中华传统经典养生术

（汉英对照）

(Chinese- English) Traditional and Classical Chinese Health Cultivation

Chief Producer　Li Jie	总策划　李　洁
Chief Compilers　Li Jie Xu Feng Xiao Bin Zhao Xiaoting	总主编　李　洁　许　峰　肖　斌　赵晓霆
Chief Translator　Han Chouping	总主译　韩丑萍
English Language Reviewer　Lawrence Lau	英译主审　芬伦斯·刘

易

筋

经

Yi Jin Jing (Sinew-Transformation Classic)

编著　倪青根
Compiler　Ni Qinggen

翻译　韩丑萍
Translator　Han Chouping

上海科学技术出版社
Shanghai Scientific & Technical Publishers

图书在版编目（CIP）数据

易筋经：汉英对照 / 倪青根编著；韩丑萍译.
—上海：上海科学技术出版社，2015.5
（中华传统经典养生术）
ISBN 978-7-5478-2551-8

Ⅰ.①易… Ⅱ.①倪… ②韩… Ⅲ.①易筋经（古代
体育）-基本知识-汉、英 Ⅳ.①G852.6

中国版本图书馆CIP数据核字（2015）第042359号

Yi Jin Jing (Sinew-Transformation Classic)

·

易

筋

经

易筋经

编著 倪青根

上海世纪出版股份有限公司
上 海 科 学 技 术 出 版 社 出版

中国图书进出口上海公司 发行

2015年5月第1版
ISBN 978-7-5478-2551-8/R·873

顾问委员会

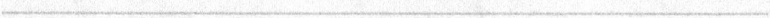

编纂委员会
Compilation Committee Members

总策划
李 洁

Chief Producer
Li Jie

总主编
李 洁 许 峰 肖 斌 赵晓霆

Chief Compilers
Li Jie　Xu Feng　Xiao Bin　Zhao Xiaoting

副总主编
孙 磊 陈昌乐 倪青根

Vice Chief Compilers
Sun Lei　Chen Changle　Ni Qinggen

总主译
韩丑萍

Chief Translator
Han Chouping

副主译
赵海磊

Vice Chief Translator
Zhao Hailei

项目资助

Acknowledgement

· 上海市新闻出版专项扶持资金项目

· 上海市中医药三年行动计划（2015—2018年）"基于〈中华气功史陈列馆〉科普教育基地为核心的〈中医气功文化平台〉建设"（项目编号：ZY3–WHJS–1–1010）

· Shanghai Press and Publication of special support funds program

· The Three-Year Action Plan for Chinese Medicine in Shanghai (2015–2018) on Construction of Qigong Cultural Platform in the Museum of Chinese Qigong History (Program No: ZY3–WHJS–1–1010)

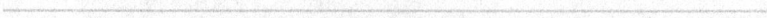

序

欣闻上海市气功研究所编写的《中华传统经典养生术》丛书即将出版,这是中华原创医学文明传播的一件盛事,特致贺忱。

中华传统养生术源远流长,其中导引术更是重要的组成部分,它先于针、灸、药、医而形成,是中华民族最早用以防治疾病、养生保健的重要方法之一。现存早期文献《庄子》《吕氏春秋》《黄帝内经》以及考古发现《引书》《导引图》中均有关于养生导引及其具体方法的记载。此后绵绵数千年的历史长河中,中华养生导引术不断丰富、发展与创新,在自我实践中形成千门万法,在去伪存真中完善理论体系。20世纪后叶,古之导引术又以现代"气功"的面目再次席卷中华大地,并享誉海内外。时至今天,中华导引术仍然以其"人天合一"的整体观思想与丰富多姿的养生导引方法独立于世界自然医药之林,滋润着人类身心世界。事实表明,中华导引术已经形成为一门博大精深的学术体系。它所研究的是人之物质基础(精)与自组织能力(神)相互关系的规律,是关于"人"——这个地球上最复杂系统达到和谐与协调的一门学问。

我和上海市气功研究所相识逾30年,该所自20世纪70年代的中医研究所开始,气功与导引就是关注、研究的重点领域;80年代中期更名气功研究所后,更是全力着眼于现代气功的研究与中华导引术的弘扬。《中华传统经典养生术》是上海市气功研究所多年来所教授养生导引术、气功功法的汇编与总结,对于帮助学习、普及推广现代导引术具有较好的价值。希望此丛书的出版,能够进一步带动当前养生导引术在海内外的健康发展,推动中华优秀文化走向世界各地。

是以为序。

林中鹏

2015年3月

It is with great pleasure that I learn the *Traditional and Classical Chinese Health Cultivation* series compiled by the Shanghai Qigong Research Institute will be published soon. This means a lot to the spread of Chinese medical civilization.

Traditional Chinese health cultivation has a long-standing and well-established history. As an important part of health cultivation practice, Dao Yin exercise was used for disease prevention and treatment as well as life cultivation before acupuncture, moxibustion and herbal medicine. The recordings of *Dao Yin* and its specific exercise methods can be traced back to the *Zhuangzi, Lü Shi Chun Qiu* (The Annals of Lü Buwei), *Huang Di Nei Jing* (the Yellow Emperor's Inner Classic) and archaeologically unearthed books such as *Yin Shu* (a book on Dao Yin) and *Dao Yin Tu* (Dao Yin Diagram). After this, the thousands of years have witnessed the enrichment, progress and innovation of Chinese *Dao Yin* practice, coupled with emergence of numerous methods and perfection of its theoretical system. In late 20th century, the ancient *Dao Yin* exercise became exceptionally popular across China in the form of 'qigong'. Today, Chinese *Dao Yin* exercise remains flourish with its holistic 'Man-Nature Unity' idea and various exercise methods that benefit both body and mind. Facts show that there is a profound academic system behind Chinese *Dao Yin* exercise. This system studies the interactions between material foundation (essence) and self-organization ability (mind). In other words, it studies the way to achieve harmony and coordination of human being—the most complex system on earth.

I've established a friendship with the Shanghai Qigong Research Institute for 30 years. Ever since its founding in 1970s as a Research Institute of Chinese Medicine, qigong and *Dao Yin* have always been the research priorities of the Institute. The focuses on qigong and *Dao Yin* have been more highlighted in 1980s when the Institute was renamed as a Qigong Research Institute. I firmly believe that the

Traditional and Classical Chinese Health Cultivation series are of great significance in popularizing modern *Dao Yin* exercise. I sincerely wish the book series can further promote *Dao Yin* exercise at home and abroad and spread excellent Chinese culture.

For this, I wrote this forward.

Lin Zhongpeng

March 2015

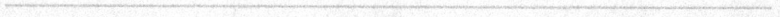

前 言

气 以 臻 道

农历乙未早春,正是上海市气功研究所创建三十周年之际,恰逢气功学术发展枯木迎春之季。在此,我们谨向海内外气功学界发出倡言——构建现代气功"气以臻道"的学术思想。

所谓"气以臻道",首先是指气功学术发展必须树立一个大方向,即中华传统文化精神的最高目标——"道";其次是指通过对"气"的感性体验与理性认知,使生命更趋向"道",与"道"合一。道者,规律、目标也;气者,方法、途径也;臻者,趋向、完善也。气-道共同构成"气以臻道"学术思想内核。其中气为实、主行,是具体之指;道为虚、主理,是抽象之喻。气因道而展,道由气而实;气以道归,道以气显;气借道而实际指归,道假气而理性论证。气功学术发展必须气、道并重,互印互证,理行一贯。两者既各尽其责、各擅其能,又有主从之别。"道"因标指形上本体而为万法归宗之源;"气"每描述形下万法而成法法生灭之流。"道"经思维抽象提炼,揭示规律、规则之理性思辨;"气"常直叙主观感觉,表述体会、觉受的感性认识。道-气,一主一从,一虚一实,构成中华气功学术思想的本质内涵。

"气以臻道"学术思想之主体是"道",是指向真理之道路,是学术文化人文精神的体现,也是先人用身心去实践生命运化规律的心得体验,古人称为"内证之学"。"道"的外延旁及"功"和"术",可以包括各种神秘现象、气功现象、特异现象,古人称为"神通法术"。当今,现代科学研究介入传统气功学术是时代进步的表现,它为我们观察生命奥秘打开了一个全新的视角。透过唯象的研究,重新激发起人类对生命的思考与敬重,重新挖掘出科技文明下的人文精神,而非单纯地将生命物质化,这才是现代科学介入传统气功的人文价值所在。

　　有鉴于此，我们倡议构建现代气功研究之"气以臻道"学术思想，让中华传统文化与现代科学携起手来，揭示生命真谛，回归大道本源。

上海市气功研究所

2015年春

Advocacy for *Qi-Dao Harmony* in Modern Qigong Practice

　　The year 2015 is a Chinese new year of yin wood sheep (*Yi Wei* in Chinese). Wood, in Chinese culture on five elements (*Wu Xing*), is connected to the season of spring. The year 2015 also marks the 30th anniversary of the founding of Shanghai Qigong Research Institute. With a strong belief that the spring of 2015 will bring new hope to qigong study, we hereby advocate the concept of 'Qi-*Dao Harmony*' for its academic advance.

　　The term *Qi-Dao Harmony* has two underlying implications. First, it implies that *dao* is the ultimate goal of traditional Chinese culture and the general orientation for academic qigong advance. Second, it implies that our lives shall combine into one with the *dao* through perception and understanding of qi. In summary, this term means to achieve and perfect *dao* through qi exercise. The 'qi' here is weighted and refers to practice. The '*dao*' here is unweighted and refers to principles. Without *dao*, qi cannot extend; without qi, *dao* cannot become weighted. Qi finds its origin in *dao* and *dao* manifests itself in qi. Qi returns to *dao* eventually and *dao* supports qi theoretically. It's essential for people in academic qigong field to pay equal attention to qi and *dao*. The two have a principal-subordinate relationship. The metaphysical *dao* is the origin of all methods. The physical qi is the practice of all methods. *Dao* is about the abstract thinking and reveals the laws and rules. Qi is about the subjective feelings and tells experience and perception. Qi and *dao* constitute the essence of academic idea in Chinese qigong.

Let's get a deeper look into the concept of *Qi-Dao Harmony*. Also known as the 'learning of internal evidence', *dao* is the way to truth: It contains humanistic spirit and physical and mental experience of our ancestors. *Dao* extends to exercise (*gong*) and a variety of magic arts including mysterious, qigong and extrasensory phenomena. Today, modern scientific qigong research offers a new insight into the mysteries of life. The phenomenological research rekindles our reflection and respect towards life and enables us to re-discover humanism from modern civilization greatly impacted by science and technology. This is the real value of scientific research on traditional qigong in this materialized world.

To this end, we advocate the academic concept of '*Qi-Dao Harmony*' in modern qigong research. We believe the combination of traditional Chinese culture and modern science can help us to reveal the truth of life and return to the origin of the great *dao*.

Shanghai Qigong Research Institute

Spring 2015

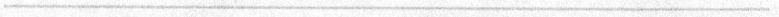

编写说明

Words from the Compilers

中华传统养生术根植于中国传统哲学、中医学和养生学，是人体自我身心锻炼的有效方法。

随着倡导"主动健康"概念日益深入人心，具有调身、调息、调心功能的中华传统养生术，以其传统的养修理论、独特的身心效果蜚声海内外，引起世人的广泛关注。但近期国内外少见中国传统养生术的书籍出版，尤其没有成套、成系列的经典养生类作品问世，更缺乏英汉对照的专业著作。

上海中医药大学上海市气功研究所研究人员在前期研究工作基础上，精选中华传统经典养生术共八种，从历史源流、功法理论、特色要领、图解动作、分解说明与具体运用几方面进行中文编纂，由上海中医药大学中医英语专业人员进行翻译。并邀请专家进行中文审稿，邀请美国友三中医药大学Lawrence Lau先生审定英文翻译。

本套丛书详细地将八种中华经典养生术以图文并茂、视频摄像的形式记录下来，配以光盘，非常方便学习与传播，尤其便于海外养生爱好者以英语来学习。

本套丛书编纂过程中，得到上海市中医药三年行动计划（2015—2018年）"基于〈中华气功史陈列馆〉科普教育基地为核心的〈中医气功文化平台〉建设"（项目编号：ZY3-WHJS-1-1010）资助。

编者

Traditional Chinese health cultivation includes a variety of body-mind exercises, which are deeply rooted in ancient Chinese philosophy and medicine.

Today, the concept of 'health initiative (an ability to achieve physical, mental and social well-being)' has become well recognized.

Traditional Chinese health cultivation exercises are attracting worldwide attention because of their unique effects in regulating the breathing, body and mind. However, there are few books in this regard, especially the classical book series. There are even fewer bilingual Chinese-English versions of these books.

Based on their previous studies, research staff at the Shanghai Qigong Research Institute compiled eight traditional and classical health cultivation exercise methods, covering their history, theoretical foundation, characteristics and key principles, illustrated movements and application. Then these contents have been translated by professional interpreters at Shanghai University of Traditional Chinese Medicine. The Chinese version was reviewed by an expert team. The English version was reviewed by Dr. Lawrence Lau at the Yo San University of Traditional Chinese Medicine.

In addition to illustrations and videos are also available for readers, especially overseas health cultivation fans to learn.

This books series have been funded by the Three-Year Action Plan for Chinese Medicine in Shanghai (2015–2018) on Construction of Qigong Cultural Platform in the Museum of Chinese Qigong History (Program No: ZY3–WHJS–1–1010).

Compilers

目 录

Table of Contents

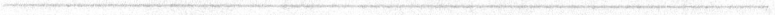

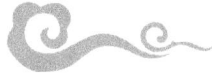

易 筋 经 ● *Yi Jin Jing* (Sinew-Transformation Classic)

源流

我国古代有多种导引术,历史悠久,易筋经是我国古代流传下来,具有强筋健骨、练气养生的导引术,是传统导引锻炼方法之一。

Numerous *Dao Yin* techniques were recorded in Chinese history. *Yi Jin Jing* is one of the traditional *Dao Yin* exercises to strengthen the tendons and bones, cultivate qi and promote health.

早在三皇五帝之前的时代,传说中的"阴康氏"部落的先民发明了一种"摔筋骨、动支节"的导引养生方法。据考证,"阴康氏"应是生活于传说中的女娲、伏羲之后,神农、黄帝之前的母系氏族部落,距今约5000年。《吕氏春秋·古乐篇》有一段记载:在阴康氏早期的生活中,地理位置不佳,天气阴冷,再加上河流缺乏管理,水道堵塞,导致人们身体不适,以筋骨酸痛、肢体活动不利,甚至关节挛缩等疾病为主。当时巫师创建了"大舞"来教人们强身健体。这就和南宋朱熹编撰的《通鉴纲目》、罗泌编撰的《路史》等所记载的"阴康氏时,水渎不疏,江不行其原,阴凝而易闷。人既郁于内,腠理滞着而多重,得所以利其关节者,乃制之舞,教人引舞以利道之,是谓大舞"是相吻合的。"大舞",也就是我们现在所说的气功导引。

Even before the era of '*Three Sovereigns and Five Emperors*'[1], ancestors in legendary *Yin Kang Shi* tribe, a matriarchal clan

---

1. A group of mythological rulers and deities from ancient China during the period circa 2852 BC to 2070 BC (In myth, the Three Sovereigns were demigods who used their abilities to help create mankind and impart to them essential skills and knowledge. The Five Emperors were exemplary sages who possessed great moral character).

society after Nüwa[1] and Fuxi[2] but before Shennong[3] and Huangdi[4] (approximately 5,000 years ago), invented a type of 'tendon-stretching and joint-moving' *Dao Yin* exercise. The *Lü Shi Chun Qiu*[5] · *Gu Le* (*Mister Lü's Spring and Autumn Annals*) states, 'during the reign of *Yin Kang Shi*, people suffered from physical discomfort, especially muscle soreness and pain, impaired movement of the limbs, and joint contracture due to geographical location, cold weather and stagnant rivers'. At that time, witches created great dance (*Da Wu*) to enhance physical health. The *Tong Jian Gang Mu* (Outline of Historical Events Retold as a Mirror for the Government) by Zhu Xi[6] and *Lu Shi* (Great History of China) by Luo Mi in the southern Son dynasty (1127–1279) also recorded, 'During the reign of *Yin Kang Shi*, flowing water in rivers stagnate, people suffered from body heaviness and joint problems. They were taught to perform some dancing movements to stretch the body. These movements were called *Da Wu* (great dance, i.e., *Dao Yin*)'.

《南华经》也有描述具体而形象的养生方法。《庄子·刻意》说:"吹呴呼吸,吐故纳新,熊经鸟申,为寿而已矣,此道(导)引之士,养形之人,彭祖寿考者之所好也。"另外湖南长沙马王堆出土的著名的《导引图》也证明了我国的传统导引术历史悠久,而易筋经的导引动作和上述也有相似之处。而巧合的是,三国

---

1. A goddess in ancient Chinese mythology best known for creating mankind and repairing the pillar of heaven.
2. A culture hero in Chinese legend and mythology, credited with creating humanity and with the invention of hunting, fishing, cooking, and (together with Cangjie) writing ca. 12,000 BCE.
3. A legendary ruler of China and cultural hero who taught the ancient Chinese not only their practices of agriculture, but also the use of herbal drugs.
4. One of the legendary Chinese sovereigns and culture heroes and now regarded as the initiator of Chinese civilization, and said to be the ancestor of all Huaxia Chinese.
5. An encyclopedic Chinese classic text compiled around 239 BCE under the patronage of the Qin Dynasty Chancellor Lü Buwei.
6. A Song Dynasty Confucian scholar who became the leading figure of the School of Principle and the most influential rationalist Neo-Confucian in China.

时期著名医师华佗所著的"五禽戏"里面的导引动作和易筋经也有相似之处。当然,从发展年代上看,五禽戏早在汉代就已十分完善和成熟,而易筋经在汉代尚没有文献记载。

The *Nan Hua Jing* (i.e. *Zhuang Zi*) recorded detailed *Dao Yin* methods. The *Zhuang Zi*[1] *Ke Ye* (Outer chapter 8 of Zhuangzi) describes, '... Breath in and out in various manners, exhale the old and inhale the new, walk like a bear and stretch their neck like a bird to achieve longevity. Such is the life favored by the scholars who practice *Dao Yin*, men who nourish the body and those who wish to live as long as Peng Zu[2]'. In addition, the *Dao Yin Tu* (Daoyin Diagram) unearthed from the Han Dynasty Tomb Mawangdui proved the long history of traditional *Dao Yin* techniques, which are similar to *Yi Jin Jing* movements. Coincidentally, *Dao Yin* movements in Five Animal Frolics (*Wu Qin Xi*) devised by Hua Tuo[3] are also similar to *Yi Jin Jing* exercise. In chronological order, the Five Animal Frolics were well established in the Han dynasty; however, there were no records of *Yi Jin Jing* at that time.

易筋经原文究竟为何人所创,历来众说纷纭。从现有文献看,大多认为易筋经、洗髓经和少林武术等为达摩所传。达摩原为南天竺国(南印度)人,公元526年来我国并最终到达嵩山少林寺,人称是我国禅宗初祖。后世流传了这样一个传说:当年,达摩祖师面壁九年后,就坐化了。被弟子们埋葬在熊耳山下,后人们不相信祖师已经坐化,打开棺木一看,却见棺木中只留有一只鞋子。后来在祖师面壁的地方,少林僧侣在修葺的时候发现

---

1. An influential Chinese philosopher who lived around the 4th century BC during the Warring States period.
2. A legendary long-lived figure in China. He supposedly lived over 800 years in the Yin dynasty (1900 to 1066 BC). He was regarded as a saint in Taoism. The pursuit of eternity drugs by supporters of Taoism was highly influenced by Peng Zu. He is well known in Chinese culture as a symbol for long life.
3. An ancient Chinese physician who is famous for his skill as a surgeon and his use of anesthesia.

了一只铁盒，没有锁，但想尽了办法都打不开，其中一个僧人想，可能是用树胶粘住了，应该用火烤，果然打开了。打开一看，内藏两部梵文薄书，一本是《洗髓经》，另一本就是《易筋经》。后来天竺僧人般刺密谛帮忙把《易筋经》翻译成了中文，达摩的传人二祖慧可则翻译了《洗髓经》，大家发现两经实为一体，《易筋经》主修外，《洗髓经》主修内。

Opinions vary on the real originator of *Yi Jin Jing*. It's now generally believed that Bodhidharma was the original ancestor of *Yi Jin Jing*, *Xi Sui Jing* (Marrow Washing Exercise) and Shaolin martial arts. Bodhidharma from India arrived in China in 526, settled at Shaolin Temple on Mount Song and became the first patriarch of Chinese Zen Buddhism. As the old legend goes, having sat facing a wall without a word for nine years, Bodhidharma passed away and was buried at the foot of Mount Xiong'er (Bear Ear) by his disciples. Later, the disciples doubted his death and opened the coffin. They only found one shoe inside the coffin. The wall Bodhidharma faced for nine years with a legacy were broken down by continual strong wind and raining. The Shao Lin monks found an iron box when they repaired the house. They tried their best to open it but in vain even though it was not locked. One monk suddenly got to understand the box of letter was stuck together by wax. When he put the iron box in fire, the wax fell off and the box was opened. There were two books written in Sanskrit, one is *Xi Sui Jing* (Marrow Washing Classic) and the other is *Yi Jin Jing* (Sinew Transforming Classic). An Indian priest named Pramati translated *Yi Jin Jing* into Chinese and Huike translated *Xi Sui Jing* into Chinese. It turned out that the two books are two parts in one: *Yi Jin Jing* to exercise the body and *Xi Sui Jing* to cultivate the mind.

《洗髓经》者，谓人之生，感于爱欲，一落有形，悉皆滓秽。

欲修佛谛，动障真如。如五脏六腑，四肢百骸，必先一一洗涤净尽，纯见清虚，方可进修，入佛智地。不由此经，进修无基，无有是处。读至此，然后知向者所谓得髓者，非譬喻也。

The *Xi Sui Jing* states, 'Through one's whole life, one always undergoes love and passion. Anyone who cannot resist on various temptations in his or her life will degenerate. Anyone who wants to gain the Prajna and the gnosis must first purely clean all of his organs and bones. Only this can he begin mortification and reach the Prajna at last. Without this process, all the sufferings he undergoes are useless and no achievement can he make. It is clear that what Bodhidharma talked about 'gaining marrow' is not in a metaphorical way'.

《易筋经》者，谓髓骨之外，皮肉之内，莫非筋连络周身，通行血气，凡属后天，皆其提挈。借假修真，非所赞勖。立见颓靡，视作泛常，曷臻极至，舍是不为，进修不力，无有是处。读至此，然后知所谓皮肉骨者，非譬喻亦非漫语也。少林寺僧修炼成效后，远游海外，二传徐鸿于海外，徐鸿三传虬髯，虬髯四传李靖。后李靖凭借易筋经建功立业。629年，大将军李靖为《易筋经》作序（时为唐贞观二载三月三日）。以528年起计，至李靖作序时隔101年，而《易筋径》已过四传。

The *Yi Jin Jing* states, 'Tendons are out of the bone and marrow but within the skin and muscles. Tendons are connected throughout the body and carry qi, blood and other things we gained after birth. So the tendon cannot be loosened or disordered. Correct exercise method can benefit the tendons. However, incorrect exercise will lead to nothing. It is clear that what Bodhidharma talked about 'gaining the skin and muscle' is neither brickbat nor in a metaphorical way'. After gaining the essence of *Yi Jin Jing* and *Xi Sui Jing*, Shaolin monks traveled overseas and first passed on to Xu Hong, who further passed on to Qiu Ran and then Qiu Ran taught Li Jing, who later became a general and was respected as a hero and held up as a model because of his highest levels of fighting ability. Li Jing wrote the preface to *Yi Jin Jing* on March 3 of the second year of Zhenguan period (629) in Tang Dynasty (618-907), which was 101 years (counting from the year 528) after passing on to 4 different people.

也有不少人认为,"易筋"之名出自道家文献,并非佛家所创的语汇。如有学者指出,在魏晋时期出现的道家求仙小说《汉武帝内传》中找到渊源。《汉武帝内传》已有"一年易气,二年易血,三年易精,四年易脉,五年易髓,六年易骨,七年易筋,八年易发,九年易形"的记载,并记载有汉朝名臣东方朔所描述的"三千年一伐毛,三千年   洗髓"等神话,这大概就是"易筋经""洗髓经"名称的由来。在宋代学者张君房所撰的道教类书《云笈七签·延陵君修真大略》中已有"易髓"、"易筋"的说法,在《云笈七签·茅山贤者服内气诀》也有相应记载:"所谓易者,能易精易形也,常法能爱精,握固,闭气,吞液,则气化为血,血化为精,精化为液,液化为骨,常行之不倦,为之一年易气,二年易骸,三年易血,四年易骨,八年易发,九年易形,十年成道……"可见,以"易"为修炼核心和鲜明手段的锻炼方法,在宋代就已经广为流传。在这里表述了道家练气求长生的一种理想。所以"易筋"原属道家思想,以及《易筋经》第一次出现时,是与清代凌延堪所著《校礼堂文集·与程雨仲书》中提到的天台紫凝道人有关,紫凝道人可能是在易筋经发展过程中起到推动作用的关键人物,或是易筋经修炼的有成就者。因此可以推断《易筋经》实为道家功法,与达摩祖师是没有什么关系的。

Some scholars argue that *Yi Jin* is not a Buddhist term but (sinew transformation) originated from Daoist literature. For example, the *Han Wu Di Nei Zhuan* (Biography of Emperor Wu of the Han Dynasty), a Daoist book in the Wei and Jin period

(220-589) records that, 'First year change the chi, second year change the blood, third year change the vessels, fourth year change the muscles, fifth year change the marrow, sixth year change the tendon, seventh year change the bone, eighth year change the hair, ninth year change the form, and from here longevity extends to many years, and there it is called immortal human being'. The myth described by Dongfan Shuo (a scholar-official in the Han dynasty) of 'changing the skin hair in 3,000 years and washing the marrow in 3,000 years' was also recorded and thought to be the origin of *Yi Jin Jing* and *Xi Sui Jing*. 'Marrow transformation' and 'sinew transformation' was also mentioned in the *Yun Ji Qi Qian Yan Ling Jun Xiu Zhen Da Lüe* (Seven Slips from a Cloudy Satchel) compiled by scholar-official Zhang Junfang in the Northern Song dynasty. The *Yun Ji Qi Qian Mao Shan Xian Zhe Fu Nei Qi Jue* (Pithy Formula for Ingestion of Internal Qi by a Sage at Mount. Mao, Seven Slips from a Cloudy Satchel) states, 'Transformation here means change of essence and form. Regular exercise of firm gripping, breathing and saliva swallowing can transform qi into blood, transform blood into essence, transform essence into humors and transform humors into bones. Over time, first year change the chi, second year change the blood, third year change the vessels, fourth year change the muscles, fifth year change the marrow, sixth year change the tendon, seventh year change the bone, eighth year change the hair, ninth year change the form, and the tenth year achieve the *Dao*'. Evidently, exercise focused on 'transformation' was associated with the Daoist idea of 'achieving longevity' and quite popular in the Song dynasty. Consequently, sinew transformation is contained in Daoist idea. The first emergence of *Yi Jin Jing* was related to *Tian Tai Zi Ning Dao Ren* (a Daoist priest) mentioned in the *Xiao Li Tang Wen Ji Yu Cheng Yu Zhong Shu* (A Letter to Cheng Yu-zhong, Collected

Works of Ling Yan-kan) by Ling Yan-kan in the Qing dynasty (1644–1912). This Daoist priest might have practiced *Yi Jin Jing* himself or played a key role in promoting its development. As a result, it can be deduced that Yi Jin Jing is actually a Daoist exercise and has nothing to do with Bodhidharma.

但不可否认和忽视的是在易筋经流传中，少林寺僧侣起到了重要作用。根据史料记载，达摩所传禅宗主要以河南嵩山少林寺为主。由于禅宗的修持大多以静坐为主，坐久则气血瘀滞，须以武术、导引术来活动筋骨。因此，六朝至隋唐年间，在河南嵩山一带盛传武术及导引术。少林寺僧侣也借此来活动筋骨，习武健身，并在这个过程中不断对其进行修改、完善、补充，使之成为一种独特的习武健身方式。最终定名为"易筋经"，并在习武僧侣中秘传。上述的传说有·定的真实性。

However, it's undeniable and non-ignorable that Shaolin monks played a significant role in passing down *Yi Jin Jing*. According to historical records, the Chan (Zen) Buddhism is mainly based in Shaolin temple in Mount. Song, Henan Province. Since monks there sit for long period of time, long-time sitting can cause qi stagnation and blood stasis, it's necessary to stretch their muscles and tendons by martial arts or *Dao Yin* movements. Martial arts and *Dao Yin* movements were therefore widespread in Shaolin temple between the Six Dynasties (229–589) and Sui-Tang (581–907) period. Through continuous modification, perfection and supplementation, Shaolin monks named these movements *Yi Jin Jing* and secretly spread among monks who practice martial arts.

自古以来，《易筋经》与《洗髓经》并行流传于世，并有《伏气图说》《易筋经义》等其他名称。《易筋经》中第一势图说即韦驮献杵。"韦驮"是佛教守护神，唐初才安于寺院中。因此，易筋经传承了我国秦汉方仙道的导引术，被少林寺僧侣改编于唐宋年间，经过多年的演绎与摸索，至明代开始流传于社会，应该是有历史依据的。

The *Yi Jin Jing* was passed down along with *Xi Sui Jing*. They are sometimes known as *Fu Qi Tu Shuo* (Illustrated Breathing Exercise) or *Yi Jin Jing Yi* (Explanations of Sinew-Transformation Exercise). The first movement in *Yi Jin Jing* is Wei Tuo Presenting the Pestle. Wei Tuo, a devoted guardian of Buddhist monasteries who guards the Buddhist teachings was placed in temple in early Tang dynasty (618–907). In summary, Yi Jin Jing was developed from *Dao Yin* movements in Qin-Han period (221 BC—220 AD), modified by Shaolin monks in Tang and Song (960–1279) dynasties and became popular in the Ming dynasty (1368–1644).

总而言之，传统易筋经从宗教、武功、中医、阴阳五行学说等方面对功法进行阐述，并且形成了不同流派，也有各自的特点，有些湮灭在了历史的长河中，有些一直流传至今。

Traditional *Yi Jin Jing* elaborates exercise methods from multiple perspectives (religion, martial arts, Chinese medicine and theories of yin, yang and five elements). There are different schools of *Yi Jin Jing*. Some survived until the present day, but some are long lost.

本书所阐述的易筋经传承了传统易筋经的理念与方法，侧重于中医传统养生，以站桩为主，结合导引术，性命双修，专气致柔，运气于奇经八脉，动作舒缓，刚柔相济，由浅入深，深入浅出，呼吸自然，不着意于意念导引，常年练习可以疏通经络，调理阴阳，振奋精神，强健身体，祛病延年。特别适合于体弱多病之人，即使一羸弱小儿亦可成健壮之体。

The *Yi Jin Jing* exercise in this text focuses on the concept and methods of health cultivation. It mainly involves *Zhan Zhuang*, incorporates *Dao Yin* movements and aims to cultivate innate nature and life endowment. Instead of using mental intent to guide physical exercise, it circulates qi among the eight extraordinary meridians through slow gentle movements and natural breathing. Persistent exercise can unblock meridians, regulate yin and yang, activate spirit, strengthen the body, remove diseases and achieve longevity. It is especially good for those with a weak constitution, including children.

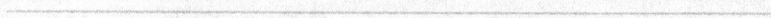

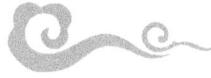

易 筋 经 · *Yi Jin Jing* (Sinew-Transformation Classic)

Theoretical Foundation

理
论
基
础

练功无外乎练精、练气、练神。各种有效的功法各有巧妙不同，易筋经也不例外。

Just like other exercise methods, *Yi Jin Jing* also cultivates essence, qi and spirit.

清 虚 与 脱 换
Into and Out of Tranquil

能清虚则无障，能脱换则无碍。要练功，首先要清静，清是神清，静是心静。在《大学》中有这样一句话：大学之道，在明明德，在亲民，在止于至善。知止而后有定，定而后能静，静而后能安，安而后能虑，虑而后能得。讲的是：大学的道理在于弘扬人的品德，在于使人去恶从善，在于使人达到完美的境界。知道了目标就能够志向坚定；志向坚定才能够静下心来不浮躁；静下心来才能够心安理得；心安理得才能够思虑周详；思虑周详才能够有所收获。所以练功首重心静，入定出定，易筋洗髓都以此为基础。

Into and out of tranquil are essential for qigong practice. With no confusion inside or obstacle outside, one can go into concentration and also can go out from concentration. The first thing in qigong practice to cleanse the mind. The *Da Xue* (Great Learning) (one of the 'Four Books' in Confucianism) states, 'What the Great Learning teaches is: to illustrate illustrious virtue; to renovate the people; and to rest in the highest excellence. The point where to rest being known, the object of pursuit is then determined; and, that being determined, a calm unperturbedness may be attained to. To that calmness there will succeed a tranquil repose. In that repose there may be careful deliberation, and that deliberation will be followed by the attainment of the desired end'. A tranquil mind is the foundation for sinew transformation and marrow washing.

为学日益，为道日损
Learning Every Day Increases,
while Following the Dao Every Day Decreases

人从小到大，在慢慢长大的过程中，身体在慢慢变老，欲望却越来越多，这对练功来说却是障碍，所谓洗髓即是洗涤自己的思想，减少自己的欲望。《道德经·第四十八章》曰"为学日益，为道日损；损之又损，以至于无为"。易筋即是通过一定的导引方法锻炼自己的身体，内外影响，心身合一，自然健康长寿。

From a small child to an adult, we tend to have more desires as we age. These desires can become obstacles for qigong practice. Marrow washing actually means to wash and cleanse our mind and greed. Chapter 48 of the *Dao De Jing* states, 'Learning every day increases, following the day every day decreases, decrease and further decrease until you reach the point of taking no action'. Through *Dao Yin* movements, *Yi Jin Jing* can benefit both the body and mind and achieve health and longevity.

性 命 双 修
Dual Cultivation of Innate Nature and Life
Endowment

孙思邈的《备急千金要方·养性序第一》曰："养性者，欲所习以成性,性自为善,不习无不利也。性既自善,内外百病自然不生,祸乱灾害亦无由作,此养性之大经也。"所以养性从做好事、帮助别人开始,养成这样的好习惯,在这一过程中,不断地反省自己,不断地完善自己,见贤思齐,磨掉浮躁与坏脾气,常思:发脾气是本能,控制脾气才是本事;当想:我是一个只受本能控制的野兽吗?

Sun Si-miao[1] mentioned in his *Bei Ji Qian Jin Yao Fang Yang Xing Xu Di Yi* (Essential Formulas for Emergencies Worth a Thousand Pieces of Gold), 'To nurture the innate nature, one needs to turn virtue and kindness into his or her second nature. With this second nature, one will not suffer from any diseases or disasters'. It's advisable to start with doing good deeds and helping others to cultivate your innate nature. You also need constantly reflect on and perfect yourself. Losing one's temper is often seen as an instinct, however, unlike animals, human being should have good abilities to control our behavior.

要收摄自己的心猿意马,要给自己立下规矩,要节制自己的言行。《道德经·第十二章》谓:五色令人目盲,五音令人耳聋,五味令人口爽,驰骋畋猎令人心发狂,难得之货令人行妨。可从小事做起,比如戒烟、戒酒,戒过于好斗,戒过于好色,戒过于贪婪,戒乱发脾气,戒放纵自己,戒傲慢无礼,戒疑神疑鬼,要止恶行善,勿以善小而不为,勿以恶小而为之。诗曰:"灵台无物谓之清,寂寂全无一念生。猿马牢收休放荡,精神谨慎莫峥嵘。"

It's also important to concentrate your mind and restrain your behavior. Chapter 12 of the *Dao De Jing* states, 'The five colors blind the eye. The five tones deafen the ear. The five flavors dull the taste. Racing and hunting madden the mind.

1. A famous traditional Chinese medicine doctor of the Sui and Tang dynasty, titled as China's King of Medicine for his significant contributions to Chinese medicine and tremendous care to his patients.

Precious things lead one astray. Therefore the sage is guided by what he feels and not by what he sees. He lets go of that and chooses this'. You can start by doing a small deed, for example, quitting smoking or drinking and abstaining from aggressive, amative, greedy, indulgent, arrogant and suspicious. Keep in mind that no virtue is too small and do no evil no matter how little it is.

身体分层，层层递进
Exercises the Body Layer by Layer

人的身体，内有五脏六腑，外有四肢百骸；内而精气与神，外而筋骨与肉。如脏腑之外，筋骨主之；筋骨之外，肌肉主之，肌肉之内，血脉主之；周身上下动摇活泼充实其中的，又主之于气。是故修炼之功，重在培养血气。精气神为无形之物，筋骨肉乃有形之物。如果专门培养无形而弃有形，则不可取；专门养炼有形而弃无形，更不可取。所以有形之身，必得无形之气，相倚而不相违，乃成不坏之体。设相违而不相倚，则有形者亦化而无形矣。是故炼筋，必须炼膜，炼膜必须炼气。然而炼筋易而炼膜难，炼膜难而炼气更难。先从极难、极乱处立定脚跟。

Internally, we have five-zang and six-fu organs. Externally, we have four limbs, muscles, tendons and bones. Internally, we can exercise our essence, qi and spirit. Externally, we can exercise our sinews, bones and muscles. Outside of the zang-fu organs, there are sinews and bones. Outside of the sinews and bones, there are muscles. Within the muscles, there are blood vessels. The driving force of human life is qi. As a result, qigong practice focuses on cultivating blood and qi. Essence, qi and spirit are invisible, while sinews, bones and muscles are visible. It's inadvisable to give up exercising the visible. It's more inadvisable to give up exercising the invisible. The tangible physical body relies on intangible qi; they do not conflict but mutually support each other. Eventually, the visible can transform into the invisible. You need to exercise fascia before sinew and exercise qi before fascia. It's difficult to exercise sinew, more difficult to exercise fascia and even more difficult to exercise qi. It's important to start from the most difficult exercise.

抱一涵元，培元守中

Embraces the One and Cultivates Yuan-primordial Qi

含其眼光，凝其耳韵，匀其鼻息，缄其口气，逸其身劳，锁其意驰，四肢不动，一念冥心。眼不视而魂在肝，耳不听而精在肾，舌不声而神在心，鼻不香而魄在肺，四肢不动而意在脾，务求培其元气，守其中气，保其正气。护其肾气，养其肝气，调其肺气，理其脾气，升其清气，降其浊气，闭其邪恶不正之气。勿伤于气，勿逆于气，勿忧思悲怒以损其气。使气清而平，平而和，和而畅达，能行于筋，串于膜，以至通身灵动，无处不行，无处不到。气至则膜起，气行则膜张。能起能张，膜与筋就能一齐坚固。如只炼筋不炼膜，而膜无所主；炼膜不炼筋，而膜无所依；炼筋、炼膜而不炼气，而筋膜泥而不起；炼气而不炼筋膜，而气痿而不能宣达流窜于筋络。气不能流窜，则筋不能坚固，所以要参互其用，错综其道。

During *Yi Jin Jing* exercise, it's important to keep the eyes open, listen attentively, breathe naturally, relax the four limbs and concentrate the mind. The liver opens into the eyes, the kidney into the ears, the heart into the tongue, the lung into the nose and spleen into four limbs. It's essential to cultivate yuan-primordial qi, keep the qi of the spleen and stomach and protect healthy qi. In other words, we need to protect kidney qi, nourish liver qi, regulate lung qi, harmonize spleen qi, ascend clean qi, descend turbid qi and block pathogenic qi. Worry, grief or anger may damage qi or cause qi to stagnate. With a smooth flow, qi can reach all body parts. When qi arrives, the fascia opens. When qi circulates, the fascia expands, and subsequently consolidates with the sinews. Exercise the sinews only, the fascia will fail to control; exercise the fascia only, the fascia will have nothing to depend; exercise the sinews and fascia alone, qi will fail to support the two; exercise qi alone, qi will fail to flow freely in sinews and fascia; and as a result, unsmooth flow of qi can result in weak sinews.

劲气行于膜间，上下相连

Internal Strength and Qi Circulates within Sinews

易筋以炼膜为先，炼膜以炼气为主。现在的人对肌肉有一定的认识，健身多以锻炼肌肉为主，但是对所说得膜，人们大多不清楚，不是脂膜之膜，是筋膜之膜。脂膜，是腔中物。筋膜，是骨外物也。筋联络关节，膜则包贴骸骨。筋与膜比较，膜软于筋；肉与膜较，膜劲于肉。膜居肉之内，骨之外，是包骨衬肉之物。行此功者，必使气串于膜间，护其骨，壮其筋，合为一体，在练功中，要仔细体会。

Sinew transformation (*Yi Jin*) starts with fascia and exercise of fascia starts with qi. Today, people have more knowledge about muscles but know little about fascia. Sinews join muscle to bone (including joints) and fascia surround muscles or other structures. Fascia is softer than sinews but harder than muscles. *Yi Jin Jing* exercise aims to circulate qi within fascia to protect the bones and strengthen the sinews.

天地为炉，阴阳为炭

Uses Heaven and Earth as a Stove and Yin and Yang as the Charcoal

一动一静互为根，一阴一阳之谓道。天地本乎阴阳，阴阳主乎动静。人的身体分阴阳，上下是阴阳，左右是阴阳，内外是阴阳，刚柔是阴阳，清浊是阴阳，动静是阴阳，动静合宜，气血和畅，百病不生，乃得尽其天年。如为情欲所牵，则动静违和。过动伤阴，阳必偏胜；过静伤阳，阴必偏胜。阴伤，阳无所成，阳亦伤也。阳伤，而阴无所生，阴亦伤。生生变化之机则被阻碍，要用导引之术，运定之法，以动化静，以静运动，运中有定，定中有运，合乎阴阳，顺乎五行，发其生机，神其变化。故能通和上下，阴平阳秘，精神乃治。调和阴阳，去旧生新，充实五脏，驱外感之诸邪，消内生之百病。

Movement and stillness are rooted in each other. One yin and one yang constitute what is called the *Dao*. Yin and yang are the law of heaven and earth. Movement is yang and stillness is yin. As for human body, the upper body is yang and the lower body is yin, the left side is yang and right side is yin, and the interior is yin and exterior is yang. Softness is yin and hardness is yang. The clean is yang and the turbid is yin. Balance between movement and stillness and harmony between qi and blood keep you away from disease and thus achieve longevity. Excessive physical exercise can damage yin and physical inactivity can damage yang, causing either yang predominance or yin predominance. Since yin and yang are mutually dependent, they mutually affect each other. Damage of either yin or yang can obstruct their mutual transformation. Containing movement in stillness and stillness in movement, *Dao Yin* movements follow the law of yin, yang and five elements, and can thus balance yin and yang, consolidate the five-zang organs, and remove both exogenous pathogens and internal problems.

奇经通脉络，造化于其中
Unblocks Eight Extraordinary Meridians

奇经八脉是任脉、督脉、冲脉、带脉、阴跷脉、阳跷脉、阴维脉、阳维脉的总称。其功能为沟通十二经脉之间的联系；对十二经气血有蓄积渗灌等调节作用。

The eight extraordinary meridians include Ren, Du, Chong, Dai, Yinqiao, Yangqiao, Yinwei and Yangwei Meridians. They strengthen the links between the twelve regular meridians and act as reservoirs of qi and blood for the twelve regular meridians.

任脉　任者，妊也。是人生育之本。行于腹面正中线，其脉多次与手足三阴及阴维脉交会，能总任一身之阴经，故称："阴脉之海。"任脉起于胞中，与女子妊娠有关，故有"任主胞胎"之说。

Ren means conception. Ren meridian starts from the lower abdomen (*Bao Zhong*) and is the foundation of reproduction. It travels along the midline of the abdomen and chest and crosses with Yinwei and six-yin meridians of hand and foot. Since it governs all yin meridians, it's known as the 'sea of yin meridians'.

督脉　督则作都讲，为阳脉之都纲。行于背部正中，其脉多次与手足三阳经及阳维脉交会，能总督一身之阳经，故称为"阳脉之海"。督脉行于脊里，上行入脑，并从脊里分出属肾，它与脑、脊髓、肾又有密切联系。任、督二脉在性命双修的过程中作用极大，李时珍曰："任督二脉，人身之子午也。乃丹家阳火阴符升降之道，坎水离火交媾之乡。"

Du means governance. Du meridian travels along the midline of the back and crosses with Yangwei and six-yang meridians of hand and foot. Since it governs all yang meridians, it's known as the 'sea of yang meridians'. In addition, Du meridian travels within the spine and enters the brain. Its branches are closely related to the kidney, brain and spinal cord.

Ren and Du meridians are extremely important to dual cultivation of innate nature and life endowment. Li Shi-zhen[1] believed 'Du meridian and Ren meridian are like midnight and midday, they are the pathway for yang ascending and yin descending and foundation for coordination between kidney water and heart fire'.

冲脉　上至于头，下至于足，贯穿全身，成为气血的要冲，能调节十二经气血故称"十二经脉之海"，又称"血海"。同女子的月经有关。

Chong meridian runs through the entire body. Upward, it reaches the head; downward, it reaches the bottom of the foot. Since it helps to regulate qi and blood of the twelve regular meridians, it's known as the 'sea of blood' and associated with menstruation.

---

1. Li Shi-zhen (1518—1593): One of the greatest Chinese physicians, herbalists and acupuncturists in history. His major contribution to clinical medicine was his 27-year work, which is found in his book Compendium of Materia Medica (*Ben Cao Gang Mu*).

带脉　起于季胁,斜向下行到带脉穴,绕身一周,如腰带,能约束纵行的诸脉。与诸多妇科疾病有关。

Dai meridian starts below the rib side and runs down to Daimai[1] (GB 26) and encircles the waist like a belt. It binds up meridians that travel longitudinally and is associated with many gynecological problems.

阴蹻脉、阳蹻脉　蹻,有轻健跷捷之意。有通行上下、濡养眼目、司眼睑开合和下肢运动的功能。

Qiao means light and agile. Yinqiao and Yangqiao meridians connects the upper body with lower body, nourish the eyes and dominate opening and closing of the eyes as well as movement of the lower limbs.

阴维脉、阳维脉　维,有维系之意。阴维脉的功能是"维络诸阴";阳维脉的功能是"维络诸阳"。

Wei means link or web. Yinwei meridian connects with all yin meridians and Yangwei meridian connects with yang meridians.

伏心猿，驾烈马

Controls the Capering Monkey in the Heart and Galloping Horse in the Mind

以心行气,意在导引之先。后谓驾阴阳二蹻:掌合指立,脚跟踮起,阴阳蹻通。易筋经的锻炼方法离不开运气通关。要使

---

1. An acupuncture point located directly below the free end of the eleventh rib, level with the umbilicus.

劲气通行，上下流转，则非驾阴阳二跷不可。阴阳二跷，乃水之河车，火之轮车，一身气道之枢纽。阴跷起，则后三关可直冲上顶。阳跷驾，则前三关可直贯注底。翻阴跷、翻阳跷时，气又可翻下逆上。分而言之，阴跷起于根，举于足。阳跷起于肩，驾于手。合而言之，阴阳跷皆起于足，应于手。阴跷起则任督通，阳跷驾则鹊桥、尾闾应。阴阳跷上下交应，则吸可到底，呼可至巅。上下顺逆错综变换，如意运行，辘轳转而玉环活，气道关窍无阻滞，亦无障蔽。千峰老人赵避尘曰："八脉开通却病无，全凭心意用功夫。"

Use the mind to guide qi, i.e., mental intent precedes *Dao Yin* movements. Then connect Yinqiao and Yangqiao meridians by closing the palms with fingers pointing upward and lifting the heels off the floor. Yinqiao and Yangqiao meridians are the pivot of qi passage throughout the body, like boats in a river and wheels of fire. They have to be connected to allow free flow of internal strength and qi. With qi ascending along the Yinqiao meridian, the three passes in the back [lower gate/Coccyx (Wei Lü Guan), middle gate (Jia Ji Guan) and upper gate/Jade Pillow (Yu Zhen Guan)] can be opened up and reach the top of the head. With qi descending along the Yangqiao meridian, the three passes in the front [Upper Dantian/Yintang (located at the midway between the medial ends of the eyebrows), middle Dantian/Danzhong (Ren 17: located at the level of the 4th intercostal space, midway between the nipples) and lower Dantian/Guanyuan (Ren 4: 3 cun below the umbilicus)] can be opened up and reach the bottom of the foot. Specifically, Yinqiao meridian starts from the heels and manifests on the feet, whereas Yangqiao meridian starts from the shoulder and manifests on the hands. In combination, Yinqiao and Yangqiao meridians both start from the feet and manifest on the hands. Yinqiao meridian is related to unobstructed qi flow in Du and Ren meridians, whereas Yangqiao meridian is related to connection of the Du and Ren meridians. With coordination of Yinqiao and Yangqiao meridians, the breathing can be deep down to the soles and up to the vertex. Master Zhao Bi-chen (1860-1942), the founder of *Qian Feng Xian Tian Pai* (Thousand-peak Immortal School) once said, 'Through whole-hearted exercise, you can open up eight extraordinary meridians and remove all diseases'.

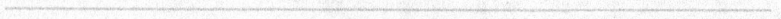

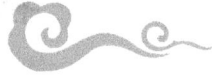

易 筋 经 · *Yi Jin Jing* (Sinew-Transformation Classic)

特色与要领

功 法 特 色
Characteristics of *Yi Jin Jing*

动作舒展，伸筋拔骨
Stretches the tendons and pulls the bones

本功法中的动作，不论是上肢、下肢还是躯干，都要求不能过分的屈伸、外展。通过适度地伸筋拔骨，循序渐进地促进身体的气血循环，改善身体的代谢过程，提高肌体的柔韧性、灵活性，达到强身健体的目的。

No matter upper limbs, lower limbs and torso are involved in movements of *Yi Jin Jing*, they cannot be excessively extended or flexed. By moderate tendon stretching and bone pulling, *Yi Jin Jing* can increase the circulation of qi and blood, improve metabolism, enable the body to be more agile and flexible and thus strengthen the body.

柔软轻灵，刚柔相济
Gentle and vigorous movements

本功法是在传统"易筋经"动作的基础上，增加了基础功法，是本套功法的重要组成部分，也是由弱到强的重要过程。通过肢体动作的变化和停顿，展现出整套功法的精髓，整个过程清晰、柔和、协调。动作速度，应均匀缓慢地移动身体或身体局部。动作相对放松,用力圆柔而轻盈,不使蛮力,不要僵硬,刚柔相济。

Based on traditional *Yi Jin Jing* practice, this exercise supplemented basic movements. Through pauses and changes of body positions, these movements can embody the essence of *Yi Jin Jing*. They are gentle, coordinated, vigorous, and performed in a slow constant speed. It's also important to relax the body, not to use strenuous exertion and combines softness with hardness.

注重腰腿,整体练习
Focuses the waist and leg

《道德经 · 第三章》中:虚其心,实其腹。即指上虚下实之意。《太极拳论》描述,其根在脚,发于脚,主宰于腰,形与手指,由脚而腿而腰,总须完整一气。故本功法的主要运动是以腰腿为主,从下而上的脊柱屈伸运动,进而带动内脏的运动,甚至进而改变骨髓的活力,达到易筋、易脏、易髓的目的。在松静自然、形神合一中完成动作,达到改变自身的目的。

Chapter 3 of the *Dao De Jing*[1] states, 'the wise therefore rule by emptying their mind and stuffing their bellies, by weakening their ambitions and strengthening their bones', indicating a cleansed mind and weighted (solid) body. The *Tai Ji Quan Lun* (Tai Ji Quan Treatise) by Wang Zong-yue states, 'the motion should be rooted in the feet, generated from the legs, directed by the waist and manifested through the fingers. All these movements are done as an integrated whole'. Through movements of the waist and legs as well as flexion and

---

1. Also simply referred to as the Laozi, is a Chinese classic text. According to tradition, it was written around 6th century BC by the sage Laozi.

extension of the spine in relaxation and tranquil, this exercise can work on the internal organs, change the bone marrow, thus transform sinew and marrow and eventually transform and improve oneself.

功 法 要 领
Essential Principles of *Yi Jin Jing*

练功要领,是指功法基本要求,是影响练功效果的原因之一。

Essential principles are basic requirements of qigong practice and are closely associated with the exercise results.

松静自然
Relaxation and tranquil

放松与清静是基本要求,也是最基本原则。《道德经·第四十五章》曰"清静以为天下正"。

Relaxation and tranquil are essential to qigong practice. Chapter 45 of the *Dao De Jing* states, 'Serenity and tranquil give the correct law to all under heaven'.

所谓自然,是指法归自然,即意念、呼吸、肢体的活动等都要自然。人法地,地法天,天法道,道法自然。精神应集中,但不应强调意守。因而练功中的自然是要做到勿忘、勿助、勿贪、勿求。

It's advisable to concentrate, breathe and conduct body movements naturally. Man follows the ways of Earth, Earth follows the ways of Heaven, and Heaven follows the ways of the

Dao. However, the Dao is a way unto itself. Concentrate but do not force yourself during qigong practice. Follow the principles of 'do not forget or hasten and do not induce or pursue'.

松静自然是练功的最基本要领,而松静最终要归于自然。所以,强调动作姿势的准确性极其重要。

An accurate posture is crucial to relaxation and tranquil.

动静结合,练养相兼
Combined motion with stillness and exercise with rest or nutrition

动则生阳,静则生阴,各有所属。动中有静,静中有动。故动与静的有机结合,可以相互促进,这样有利于内气的运行,又能提高练功效果。

Physical exercise generates yang and static meditation generates yin. There is static meditation in physical exercise and vice versa. A perfect combination of the two can benefit flow of internal qi and increase the exercise result.

练养相兼,是指练功与合理休养、调养并重,即练中有养,又练又养,这对于体质较差及慢性病患者尤其重要。养另一方面是指在进行一系列的内部锻炼后必须修整、调护,休养生息,而不应无休止地练。初学者练功后可能会觉得疲劳,因此适当增加一些营养甚至药物也是调养之意,同时要注意饮食、四时节气,六淫邪气,避之有时。日积月累,气血旺盛,终有所成。

It's also important to combine exercise with rest or nutrition, especially for those with a weak constitution or chronic conditions. It's essential to rest and recuperate after a series of exercises. Beginners often feel exhausted after exercise, and therefore need nutritious food or medicine. In addition, it's advisable to adapt to seasonal changes and avoid six pathogenic factors. Over time, *Yi Jin Jing* exercise can help to supplement qi and blood and improve your health.

循序渐进，持之以恒
Step-by-step exercise and perseverance

循序渐进，持之以恒，是指练功最好能坚持不懈。传统功法的实践性都很强，没有靠嘴巴和想法就能获得要义和功效的，纸上得来终觉浅，要知此事须躬行。经过长期练习，才能求得效果。"功练千遍，其效自见" 即是此意。

Perseverance is needed in qigong practice. What's learned from the books is superficial, and it's necessary to have it personally tested. Practice is the only way to get its essence.

1. 头颈：头正颈松
1. Head and neck: Head upright and neck relaxed

头部要正直。身体也要中正，一些功法中常提到 "头如悬" 或 "悬顶"，即是说头顶正中好像被一根线向上牵着，这样头部自然就正直了。

It's necessary to keep the head and body upright, like a threadlike string pulling the top of the head.

2. 上肢：沉肩坠肘

2. Upper limbs: Shoulder relaxed and elbows dropped

首先是肩一定要放松，要自然垂下来，绝对不要耸肩。

The shoulders shall be completely relaxed and open. Do not shrug the shoulder.

坠肘是指两肘下垂，不可用力。松肩不仅是肩膀的放松，而且要顺势松到肘。整个肩臂放松了，坠肘就可以自然形成。

Drop the elbows naturally. When you completely relax the shoulder and arms, you can naturally drop the elbows.

另外，在站桩时，有虚腋的要求，即腋下像夹着个鸡蛋，过松，蛋落，过紧，蛋碎。

In addition, it's necessary to tighten the armpit like holding an egg there (the egg may fall down to the floor if it's not firmly held; the egg may break if it's too firmly held).

3. 胸背：含胸拔背

3. Chest and back: Tuck the chest in and pull up the back

含胸与拔背的操作是同时的，拔的意思是挺拔而不弯曲，身体正直不弯曲即不前屈也不后仰之意。

The chest is depressed naturally inward and simultaneously the back is pulled up (tall, straight and upright).

4. 腰胯：沉腰坐

4. Waist and crotch: The waist sunk and crotch lowered

无论是站式还是坐式，沉腰坐胯十分重要。坐胯是胯部要收紧，向后，向下坐，同时腰反而要放松。

Sinking the waist and lowering the crotch is equally important in sitting or standing postures. Lowering the crotch means to tighten the crotch backward and downward. At the same time, the waist needs to be relaxed.

5. 下肢：轻灵安稳

5. Lower limbs: Light and agile

姿势站立稳固，身体要轻灵。

With a solid standing posture, your body needs to feel light and agile.

另外，站桩时下肢（连带整个身体）并非完全挺直不动。一般情况下，有些微微的晃动，这不是站立不稳，而是为了站立的更稳。微有晃动的站立不断地调整身体，使之更好地体会到整体的含义。

In addition, the lower limbs (or the entire body) are not necessary static during *Zhan Zhuang*. Generally, slight wobbling helps to a more stable standing.

练功时要持之以恒，关键在于"恒"字，正所谓千招会不如一招熟。要循序渐进，忌急于求成。要用意不用力，既不刻意追求，又不流于疏散。要心胸开阔，杂念袭来如浮云，了无所依，又如洪炉大冶，可使万念成灰。要循规守矩，但又不拘泥于形式，即"明规矩而守规矩，脱规矩而合规矩"。不依规矩则易生偏差，拘泥于形式则易致拘束、紧张，要用心去思考，用心去求证。运动量要因人、因病、因时、因地制宜，原则上行功者应感到轻松、自然、呼吸平静，如此由浅入深，始终使练功阶段处于轻松愉快、呼吸平静的过程，功后心境怡然，精力充沛，逐步达到预期效果。

For qigong practice, it's important to persevere, practice step by step and use your mind instead of force. It's also essential to remove distracting thoughts and not to pursue a fast success. What's more, it's advisable to follow the rules but not rigidly adhere to them. Not following the rules may cause deviation; however, rigidly adhering to rules may cause restrain or tension. Just use you mind to think and prove. Amount of exercise varies greatly from person to person. In principle, you should feel relaxed and at ease during exercise and refreshed and energetic after exercise.

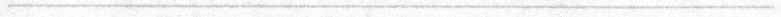

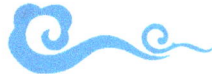

易 筋 经 • *Yi Jin Jing* (Sinew-Transformation Classic)

Movements of *Yi Jin Jing*

功法操作

基 础 操 作

Basic posture

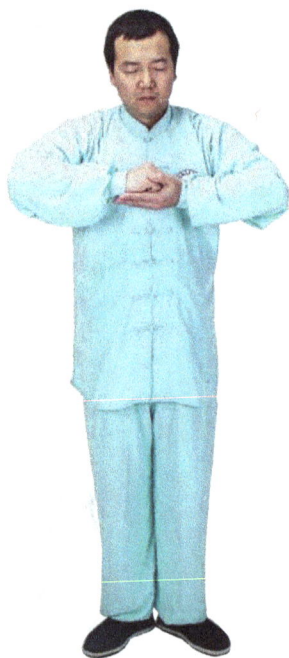

基础图1-1　Basic Posture 1-1

　　两足开立，脚跟并拢，两脚尖成八字形，然后两手缓缓上抬，两脚同时缓缓立起，屈肘于胸前，合掌。

　　Stand upright with separated feet, put the heels together and turn toes of both feet outward. Slowly lift the hands and feet, flex the elbows in front of the chest and close the palms.

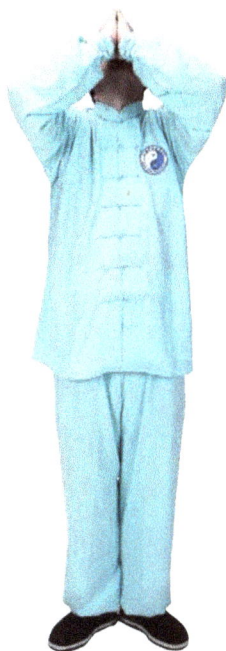

将脚跟慢慢放平立定，缓缓将头向后倒仰，朝天合掌，以仰面朝天为度。

Put the heels back to the floor, slowly lean the head backward (with the face towards the sky) and close the palms.

基础图1-2　Basic Posture 1-2

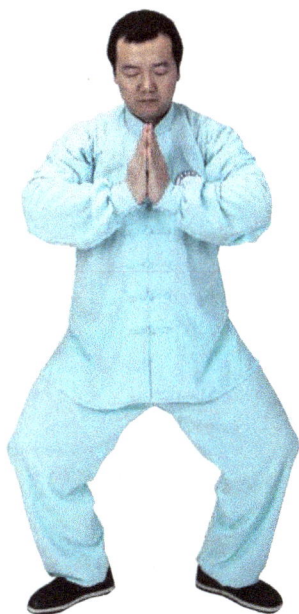

将脚跟离地，下身如骑马势，两脚成外八字，大腿与小腿成90°，双手合掌于胸前，上身中正，下坐。

Lift the heels off the floor, make the lower body a horse riding posture and turn the toes of both feet outward, forming approximately 90° between the thigh and lower leg. Close the palms in front of the chest, and keep the upper body upright and lower body down.

基础图1-3　Basic Posture 1-3

具 体 操 作
Individual Movements

第一势 韦驮献杵
Movement # 1 Wei Tuo Presenting the Pestle

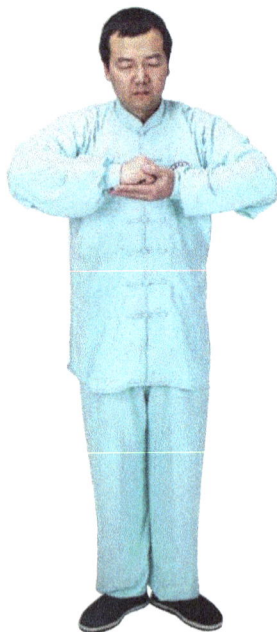

图1-1 Fig 1-1

　　两足开立,脚跟并拢,两脚尖成八字形,两臂自然下垂于体侧;身胸挺直,两目平视,定心凝神;然后两手缓缓上抬,两脚同时缓缓立起,屈肘于胸前,合掌。停立30秒至10分钟,循序渐进,量力而行。

　　Stand upright with separated feet, put the heels together, turn toes of both feet outward and drop the arms naturally to the sides. Keep the body upright, look straight ahead and cleanse the mind. Slowly lift the hands and feet, flex the elbows in front of the chest and close the palms. Stay still from 30 seconds to 10 minutes according to individualized body condition.

[诀曰]立身期正直，环拱手当胸，气定神皆敛，心澄貌亦恭。

[Tips] Keep the body upright, closes the palms in front of the chest, cleanse the mind and have a sense of respect.

[功效]调理三焦，理气和中，疏通经络，增长脚力。

[Function] This movement regulates Sanjiao, harmonize qi of the middle jiao, unblock meridians and increase the strength of the feet.

第二势　横担降魔杵
Movement # 2　Shoulder up an Evil-Banishing Pole

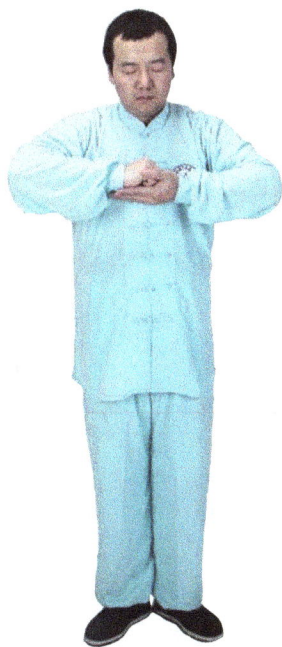

两足开立，脚跟并拢，两脚尖成八字形，两臂自然下垂于体侧；身胸挺直，两目平视，定心凝神；然后两手缓缓上抬，两脚同时缓缓立起，屈肘于胸前，合掌。

Stand upright with separated feet, put the heels together, turn toes of both feet outward and drop the arms naturally to the sides. Keep the body upright, look straight ahead and cleanse the mind. Slowly lift the hands and feet, flex the elbows in front of the chest and close the palms.

图2-1　Fig 2-1

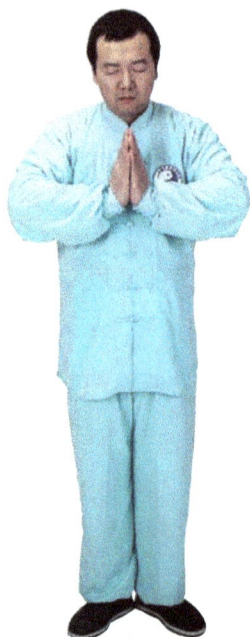

接前势，双手打开，回抱合
掌，指尖齐于鼻尖。

Further to movement # 1, open
the hands, then take back and close
the palms, making the fingertips at
the same level of the nasal tip.

图2-2　Fig 2-2

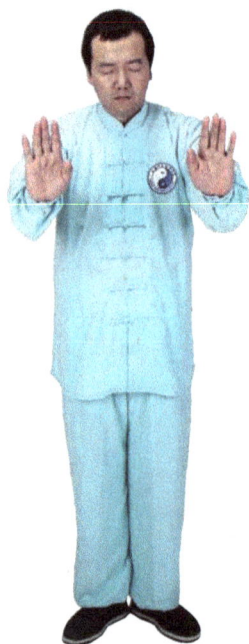

稍停一会，将手尽力向前推
出，立掌，与肩齐，两掌底与两肩
角相对。稍停一会，接着两掌回
收，平肩，掌立。

Pause for a while and then
make an effort to push forward. Keep
the palms upright at the same level
of the shoulders and let the bottom
of the palms opposite to the humeral
angles. Pause for a while, take back
the palms, square the shoulder and
keep the palms upright.

图2-3　Fig 2-3

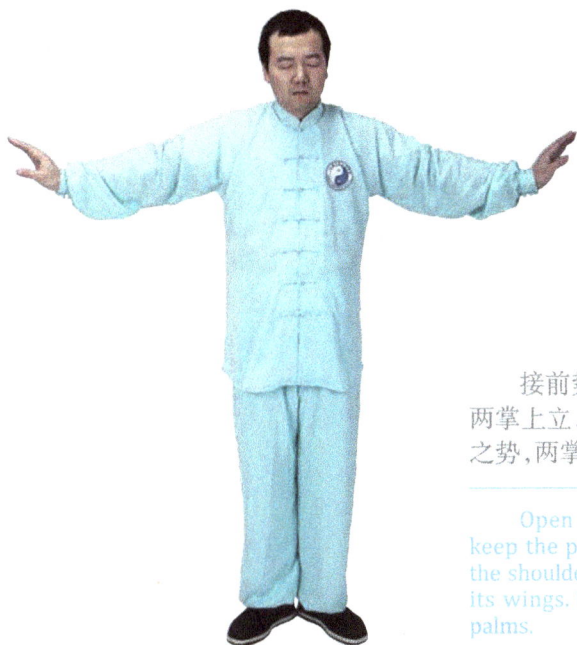

接前势，将两手向两侧撑开，两掌上立，肩膀平直，如飞鹰展翅之势，两掌缓缓撑开。

Open the hands to both sides, keep the palms upright, and square the shoulders like an eagle spreading its wings. Then slowly prop up the palms.

图2-4　Fig 2-4

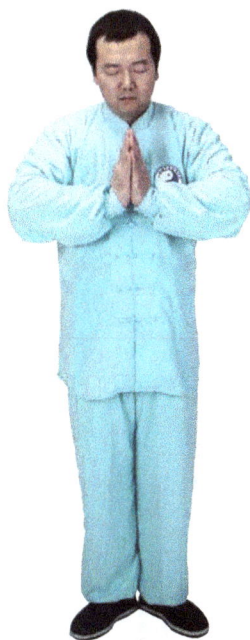

接前势，双手打开，回抱合掌，指尖齐于鼻尖。

Open the hands, then take back and close the palms, making the fingertips at the same level of the nasal tip.

图2-5　Fig 2-5

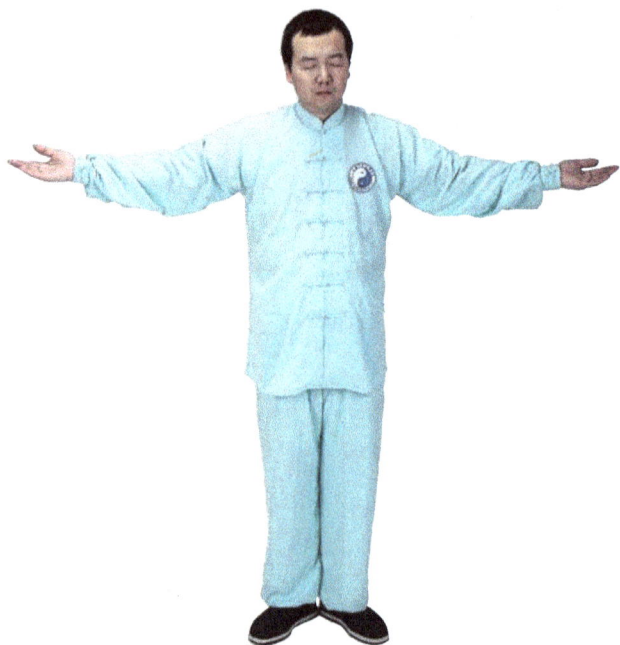

图2-6   Fig 2-6

接上式,自然呼吸,两臂由胸前向两侧平展,掌心朝上;同时两足跟提起,足尖仍着地;两目圆睁平视,心平气和。停立30秒至10分钟,循序渐进,量力而行。

Breath naturally and extend the arms from front of the chest to both sides, with palms upward. Lift the heels off the floor with toes still touching the floor. Make the eyes wide open, look straight ahead and breathe naturally. Stay still from 30 seconds to 10 minutes according to individualized body condition.

[诀曰]足指挂地,两手平开,心平气静,目瞪口呆。

[Tips] Touch the floor with the toes, open the hands, keep a natural breathing and make the eyes wide open.

[功效]宽胸理气,疏通经络,增长脚力。

[Function] This movement soothes the chest, regulates qi, unblocks meridians and increases the strength of the feet.

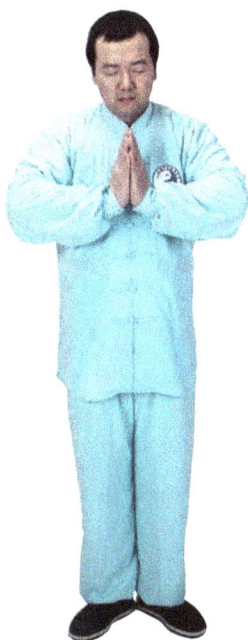

接前势，双手慢慢回抱合掌，指尖齐于鼻尖。

Slowly take back and close the palms and make the finger tips at the same level of the nasal tip.

图2-7　Fig 2-7

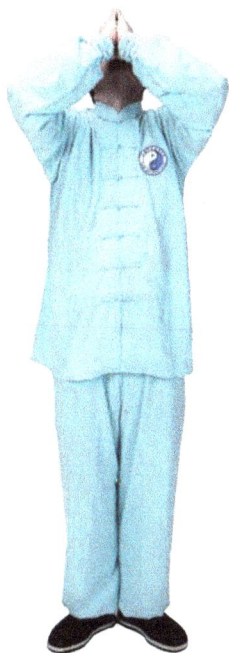

接前势，将脚跟慢慢放平立定，缓缓将头向后倒仰，朝天合掌，以仰面朝天为度。

Slowly put the heels down, make the head lean backward (with the face towards the sky) and close the palms.

图2-8　Fig 2-8

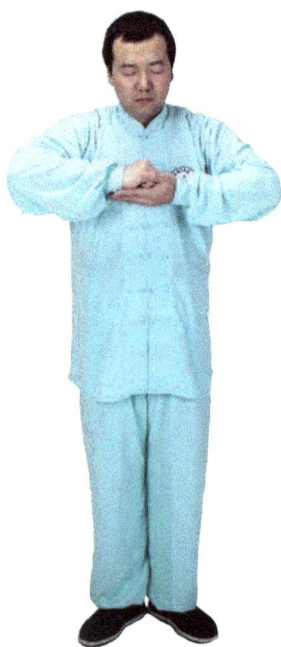

图2-9 Fig 2-9

接前势，缓缓顺势回转，返回第一势。

Slowly turn back and return to movement # 1.

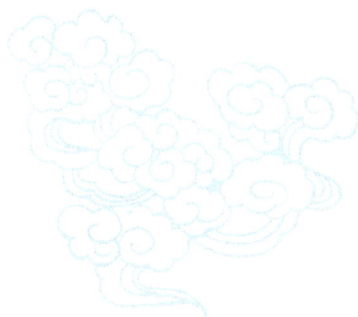

第三势　掌托天门

Movement # 3　Support the Sky with the Palms

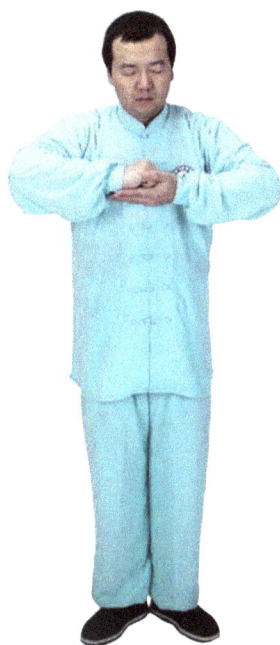

两足开立，脚跟并拢，两脚尖成八字形，两臂自然下垂于体侧；身胸挺直，两目平视，定心凝神；然后两手缓缓上抬，两脚同时缓缓立起，屈肘于胸前，合掌。

Stand upright with separated feet, put the heels together, turn toes of both feet outward and drop the arms naturally to the sides. Keep the body upright, look straight ahead and cleanse the mind. Slowly lift the hands and feet, flex the elbows in front of the chest and close the palms.

图3-1　Fig 3-1

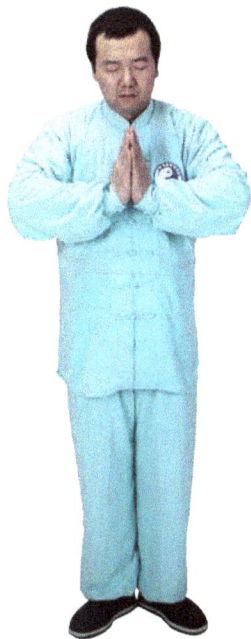

接前势，双手打开，回抱合掌，指尖齐于鼻尖。

Open the hands, then take back and close the palms, making the fingertips at the same level of the nasal tip.

图3-2　Fig 3-2

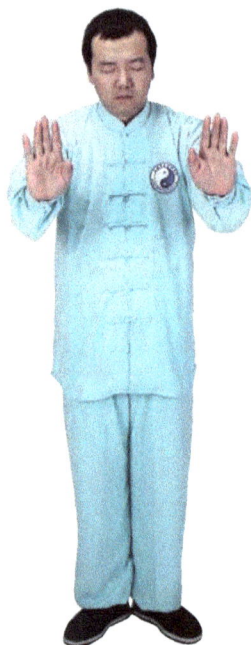

稍停一会，将手尽力向前推出，立掌，与肩齐，两掌底与两肩角相对。稍停一会，接着两掌回收，平肩，掌立。

Pause for a while and then make an effort to push forward. Keep the palms upright at the same level of the shoulders and let the bottom of the palms opposite to the humeral angles. Pause for a while, take back the palms, square the shoulder and keep the palms upright.

图3-3　Fig 3-3

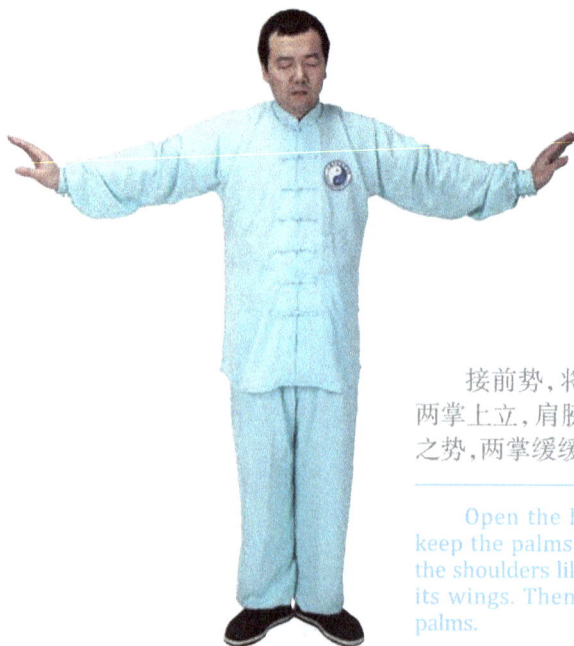

接前势，将两手向两侧撑开，两掌上立，肩膀平直，如飞鹰展翅之势，两掌缓缓撑开。

Open the hands to both sides, keep the palms upright, and square the shoulders like an eagle spreading its wings. Then slowly prop up the palms.

图3-4　Fig 3-4

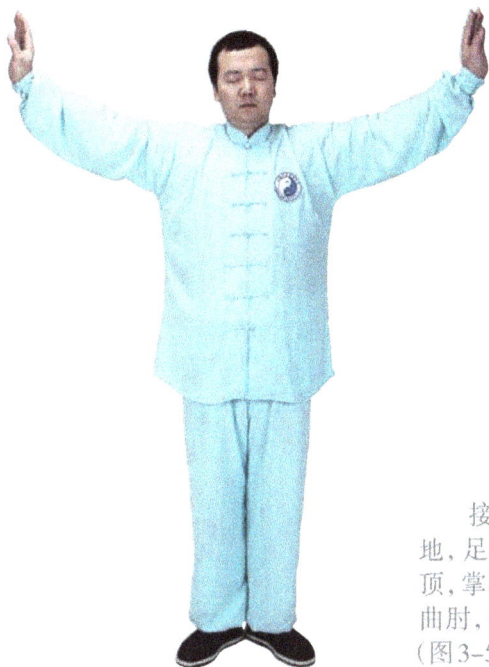

图3-5　Fig 3-5

　　接前势，两脚开立，足尖着地，足跟提起；双手上举高过头顶，掌心向上，两中指相对；沉肩曲肘，仰头，目观掌背，鼻息调匀（图3-5、图3-6）。

Separate the feet with toes touching the floor and lift the heels off the floor. Lift the hands above the top of the head, with the palms upward and two middle fingers facing each other. Drop the shoulders, flex the elbows, focus the eyes on the dorsa of the palms and breathe naturally with the nose. (Fig 3-5, Fig 3-6)

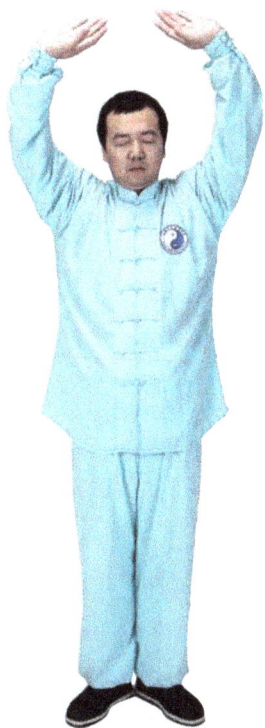

图3-6　Fig 3-6

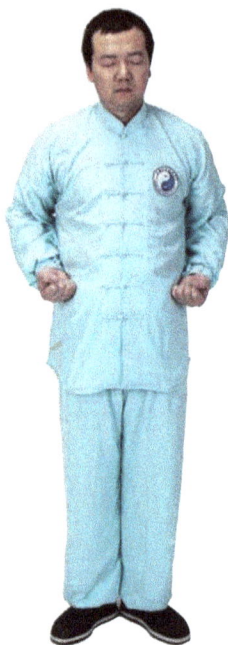

收势时，两掌变拳，拳背向前，上肢用力将两拳缓缓收至腰部，拳心向上，脚跟着地。停立30秒至10分钟，循序渐进，量力而行。

Turn the palms into fists, with the dorsa of the palms forward. Make an effort to take back the fists to the waist, with the palms upward and heels touching the floor. Stay still from 30 seconds to 10 minutes according to individualized body condition.

图3-7　Fig 3-7

［诀曰］掌托天门目上观，足尖着地立身端。力周腿胁浑如植，咬紧牙关不放宽，舌可生津将腭舐，鼻能调息觉心安。两拳缓缓收回处，用力还将挟重看。

[Tips] Lift the sky with the palms, touch the floor with the toes, do not use force from the upper limbs, touch the palate with the tongue, breathe naturally with the nose and slowly take back the fists.

［功效］调理脾胃，活血通络，增长脚力。

[Functions] This movement regulates the spleen and stomach, invigorates blood and increase the strength of the feet.

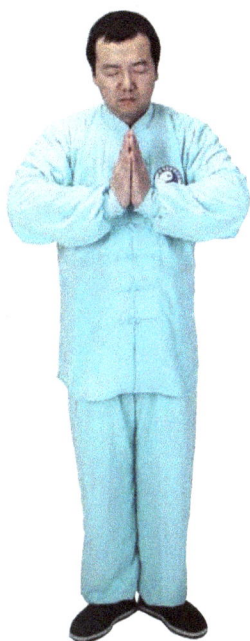

接前势，双手打开，回抱合掌，指尖齐于鼻尖。

Slowly open the hands, then take back and close the palms, making the finger tips at the same level of the nasal tip.

图3-8　Fig 3-8

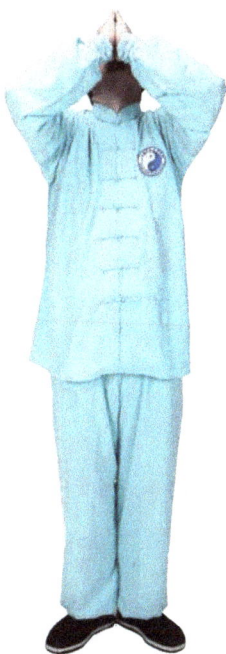

接前势，将脚跟慢慢放平立定，缓缓将头向后倒仰，朝天合掌，以仰面朝天为度。

Slowly put the heels down, make the head lean backward (with the face towards the sky) and close the palms.

图3-9　Fig 3-9

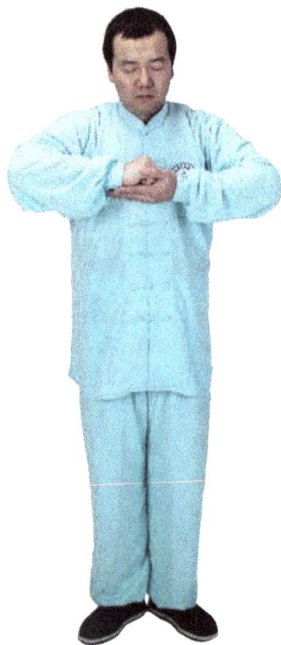

图3-10　Fig 3-10

接前势，缓缓顺势回转，返回第一势。

Slowly turn back and return to movement # 1.

第四势　摘星换斗

Movement # 4　Plucking a Star and Exchanging a Star Cluster

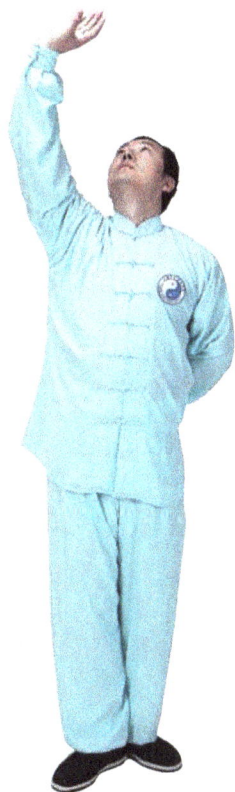

图4-1　Fig 4-1

两足跟缓缓落地,将两脚相依,站如丁字,左臂由上向下落于背后,握空心拳;同时右掌掌心朝上,掌指向左,头向右扭,目视右掌。

Slowly drop the heels to the floor, put the feet together and stand in a T-shaped position. Drop the left arm, place behind the back and make an empty fist. Turn the right palm upward, with the palm and fingers pointing towards left. Turn the head to the right and focus the eyes on the right palm.

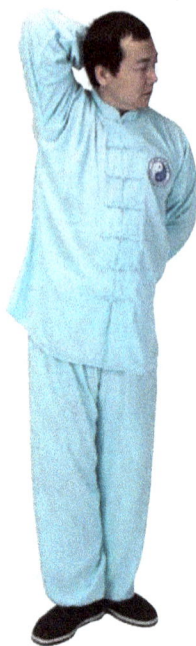

图4-2　Fig 4-2

定式后要气贯胸际，稍调呼吸，然后松右臂，缓缓向下落于背后；同时左臂由背后缓缓上举，掌心朝上，掌指向右，头向左扭，目视左掌。停立30秒至10分钟，循序渐进，量力而行。

It's advisable to soothe qi in the chest and breathe naturally. Relax, drop the right arm, place behind the back and make an empty fist. Turn the left palm upward, with the palm and fingers pointing towards right. Turn the head to the left and focus the eyes on the left palm. Stay still from 30 seconds to 10 minutes according to individualized body condition.

[诀曰] 只手擎天掌覆头，更从掌内注双眸。鼻端吸气频调息，用力回收左右侔。

[Tips] Lift the sky with one palm, focus the eyes on the palm, breathe naturally with the nose and turn to left and right alternately.

[功效] 宽胸理气，活泼肢体。

[Functions] This movement soothes the chest, regulate qi and exercise the limbs.

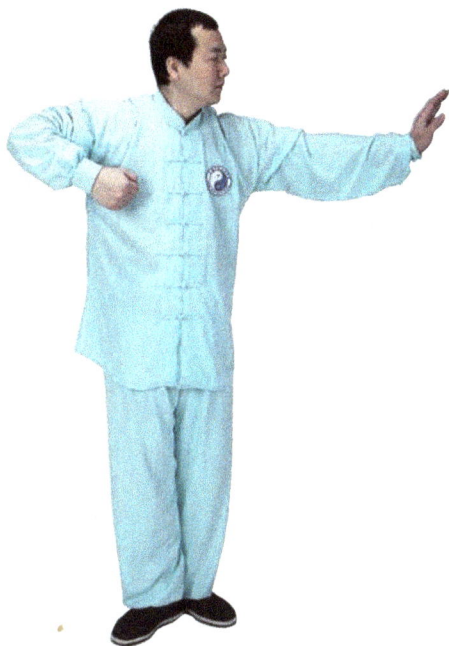

图4-3　Fig 4-3

接前势，将右手着力绕头一转，由前转后，由后顺前至右肩窝处，即将右手握拳。接前势，左手放开、平掌、顺势，向左逆撑，高与肩平，又随势收回；两脚换丁字步向左，然后立定脚跟，竖起膝腿腰脊，将左曲腕与右平掌向两边一撑，如开弓状，头向左旋，目注左掌，右曲腕与左掌相对，静心凝神，将右拳打出。

Wind the right hand around the head from front to back, and then from back to front until the right glenoid fossa. Turn the right hand into a fist. Release the left hand, make the palm flat, prop up to the left (at the level of the shoulder) and then take back. Stand in a T-shaped position and turn left, touch the floor with the heel, and straighten the knee, leg and waist. Open the flexed left wrist and flat right palm to both sides like drawing a bow. Turn the head to the left and focus the eyes on the left palm. Make the flexed right wrist face to the left palm, concentrate the mind and strike the right fist out.

右三势毕。再换左三势，其余相同。至于上身皆宜正直，不要偏倚（图4-4、图4-5、图4-6）。

Then perform the same procedure in an opposite direction. It's important to keep the upper body upright. (Fig 4-4, Fig 4-5, Fig 4-6)

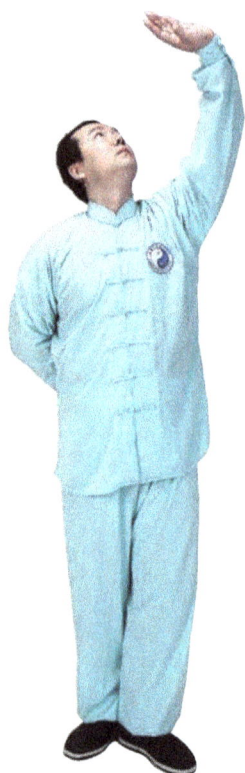

图4-4　Fig 4-4

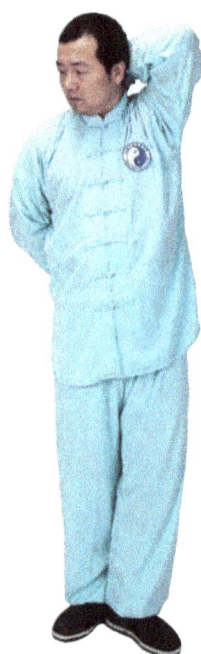

图4-5　Fig 4-5

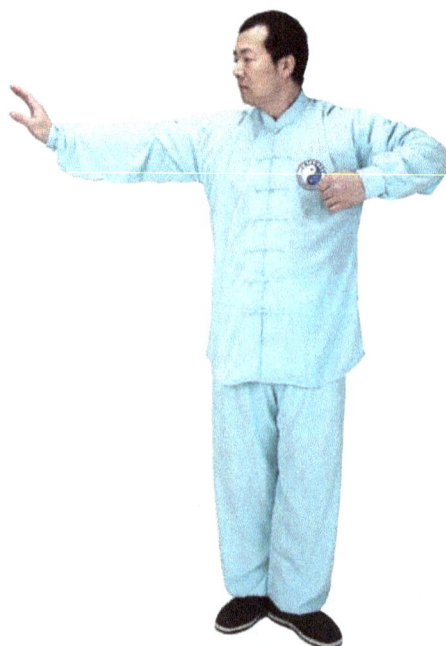

图4-6　Fig 4-6

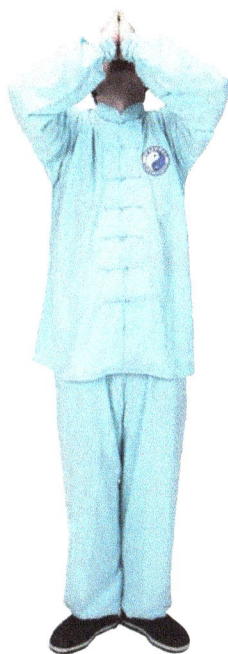

接前势，将脚跟慢慢放平立定，缓缓将头向后倒仰，朝天合掌，以仰面朝天为度。

Slowly put the heels down, make the head lean backward (with the face towards the sky) and close the palms.

图4-7　Fig 4-7

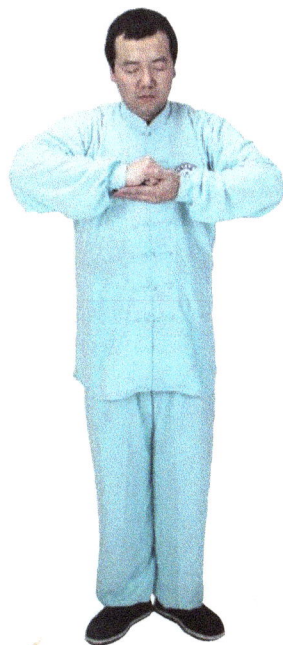

接前势，缓缓顺势回转，返回第一势。

Slowly turn back and return to movement # 1.

图4-8　Fig 4-8

第五势 倒拽九牛尾

Movement # 5 Pulling Nine Cows by Their Tails

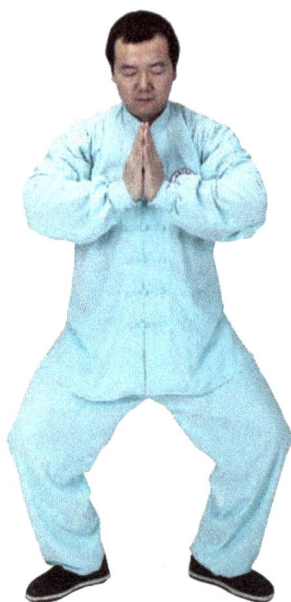

将脚跟离地，下身如骑马势，两脚成外八字，大腿与小腿成90°，双手合掌于胸前，上身中正，下坐。

Lift the heels off the floor, make the lower body a horse riding posture and turn the toes of both feet outward, forming approximately 90° between the thigh and lower leg. Close the palms in front of the chest, and keep the upper body upright and lower body down.

图5-1　Fig 5-1

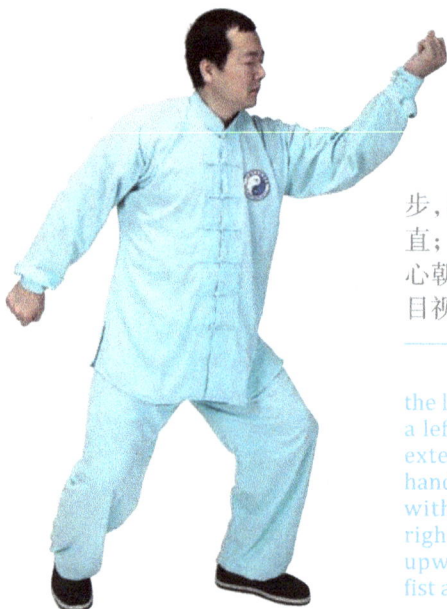

接上式，抬左脚向左侧跨一步，屈膝成左弓步。左腿屈，右腿直；同时左手由背后转至胸前，拳心朝上；右臂向后甩，拳心朝上；目视左拳。定式后静立。

Move the left foot one step to the left side, bend at the knee to form a left bow step. Flex the left leg and extend the right leg. Turn the left hand from back to front of the chest with the palm upward. Swing the right arm backward with the palm upward. Focus the eyes on the left fist and stand still.

图5-2　Fig 5-2

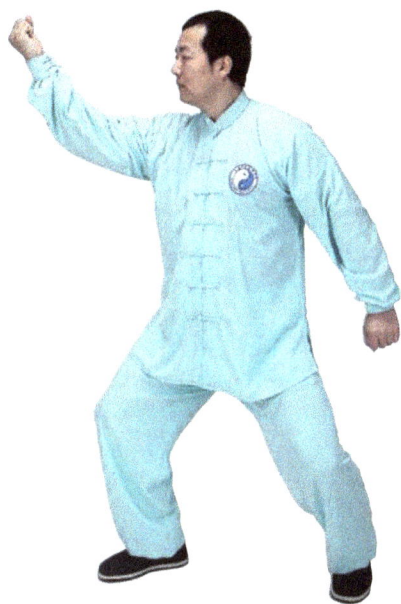

而后，左右腿势互换，成右弓步，同时右拳由背后缓缓伸向身前，左拳由向前缓缓移向背后，目视右拳。停立30秒至10分钟，循序渐进，量力而行。

Then change the position of the left and right leg and form a right bow step. Slowly extend the right fist from back to the front of the body, move the left fist from front to back and focus the eyes on the right fist. Stay still from 30 seconds to 10 minutes according to individualized body condition.

图5-3　Fig 5-3

[诀曰] 两腿后伸前屈，小腹运气空松；用力在于两膀，观拳须注双瞳。

[Tips] Flexion and extension of the legs, enable qi to move in the lower abdomen, use force from the arms and focus the eyes on the fists.

[功效] 调整体质，伸筋拔骨，疏通经络，增长体力。

[Functions] This movement regulates the body constitution, stretches the tendons, pulls the bones, unblocks meridians and increases physical strength.

接前势，将手、脚、头、身换右。其余相同。停立30秒至10分钟，循序渐进，量力而行。

Perform the same procedure in an opposite direction (right side). Stay still from 30 seconds to 10 minutes according to individualized body condition.

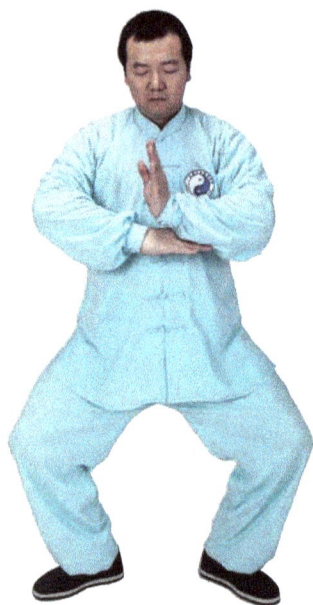

接前势，收回手脚，端正头身，下身脚尖点地如骑马状；左肘关节屈转，平胸立掌；右肘关节屈转，平掌放于立掌下，掌背朝上。

Take back the hands and feet and keep the head and body upright. Touch the floor with the toes like riding a horse. Flex the left elbow and make the chest flat and palm upright. Flex the right elbow and place the flat palm underneath the upright (left) palm, with the dorsum of the palm upward.

图5-4　Fig 5-4

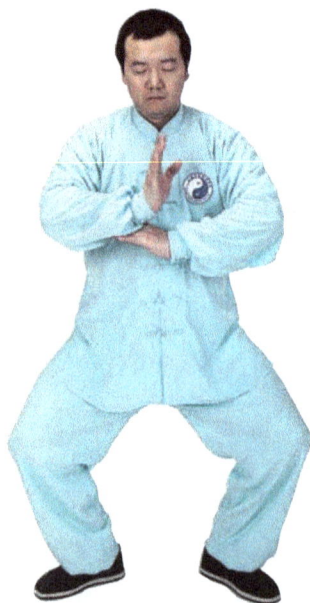

此势就前势，左掌换如右，右掌换如左，其余相同。

Perform the same procedure using the left palm and right palm alternately.

图5-5　Fig 5-5

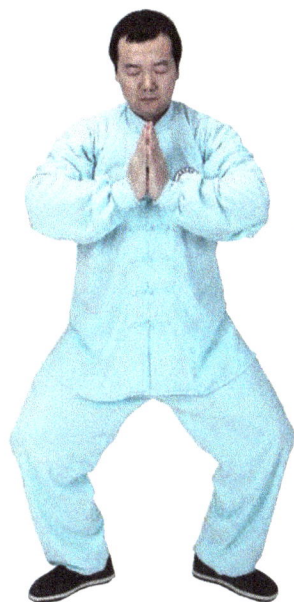

接前势，双手打开，再缓缓
收回到胸前。

Open the hands and slowly take
back to the front of the chest.

图5-6　Fig 5-6

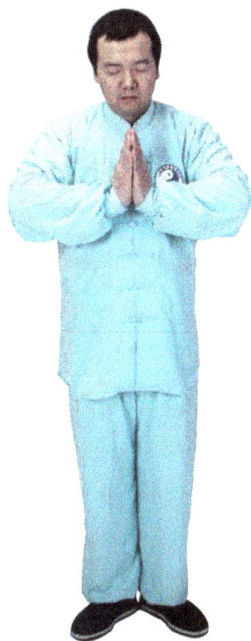

接前势，缓缓起立，两脚收回，
仍脚尖着地，两掌不变。

Slowly stands up and take back
the feet, still keeping the palms and
touching the floor with the toes.

图5-7　Fig 5-7

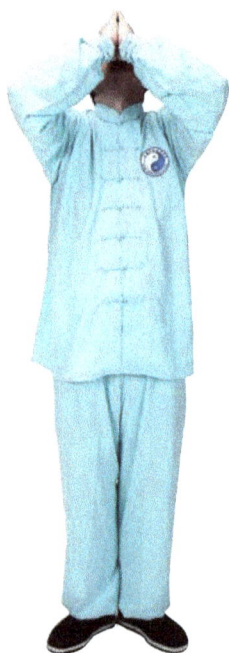

接前势，将脚跟慢慢放平立
定，缓缓将头向后倒仰，朝天合
掌，以仰面朝天为度。

Slowly put the heels down, make
the head lean backward (with the face
towards the sky) and close the palms.

图5-8　Fig 5-8

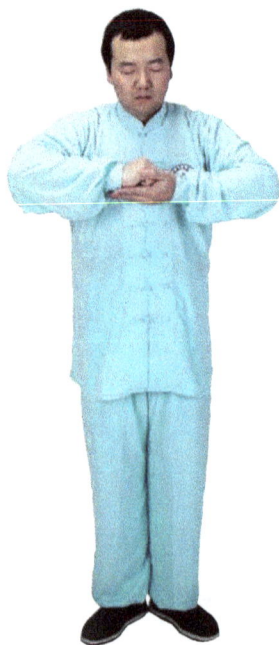

接前势，缓缓顺势回转，返回
第一势。

Slowly turn back and return to
movement # 1.

图5-9　Fig 5-9

第六势 出爪亮翅

Movement # 6　Displaying Paw-Style Palms like a White Crane Spreading Its Wings

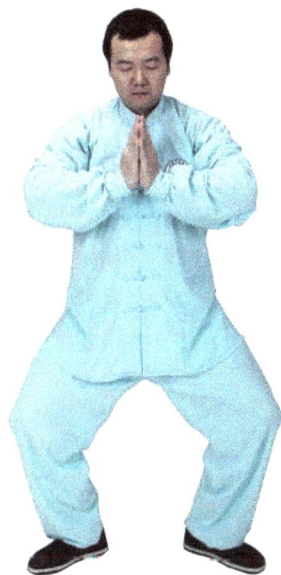

将脚跟离地，下身如骑马势，两脚成外八字，大腿与小腿成90°，双手合掌于胸前，上身中正，下坐。

Lift the heels off the floor, make the lower body a horse riding posture and turn the toes of both feet outward, forming approximately 90° between the thigh and lower leg. Close the palms in front of the chest, and keep the upper body upright and lower body down.

图6-1　Fig 6-1

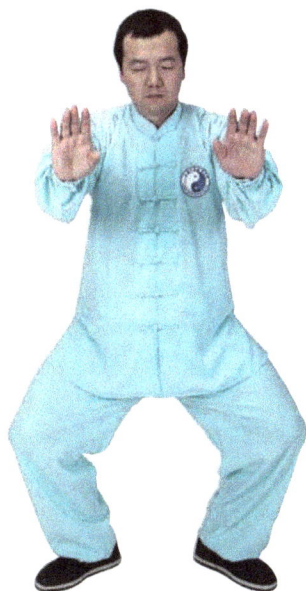

接上式，收左脚缓落于右脚后半步，两脚碾地，使两腿成排步，同时两拳收于腹侧；然后变掌一齐向胸前缓缓推出，同时两腿缓缓微蹲，掌心向前，掌指向上；圆睁双目，全身放松；随之两掌变拳，收回腹际两侧，掌心向上，然后再变掌向前推出。依此法反复。停立30秒至10分钟，循序渐进，量力而行。

Take back the left foot to half a step posterior to the right foot, touch the floor with the feet (forming a position of 'standing at attention') and take back the fists to the ventral sides of the body. Turn the palms and slowly push forward and slightly flex the legs with the center of the palms forward and fingers upward. Make the eyes wide open, relax the body, turn the palms into fists and take back to both sides of the body. Make the palms upward, turn the palms and push forward. Repeat this and stay still from 30 seconds to 10 minutes according to individualized body condition.

图6-2　Fig 6-2

Yi Jin Jing (Sinew-Transformation Classic) · 易筋经

63

功法操作 · Movements of *Yi Jin Jing*

［诀曰］挺身兼怒目，推手向当前；用力收回处，功须七次全。

[Tips] Straighten the back with glaring eyes, push the hands forward, make an effort to take back and repeat 7 times.

［功效］调理肺气，疏通经络，增长体力。

[Functions] This movement regulates lung qi, unblocks meridians and increases physical strength.

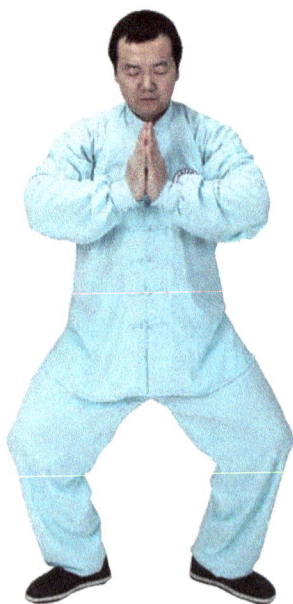

图6-3　Fig 6-3

接前势，缓缓将双手收回，到胸前合掌，返回第一势。

Take back and close the hands in front of the chest, return to movement # 1.

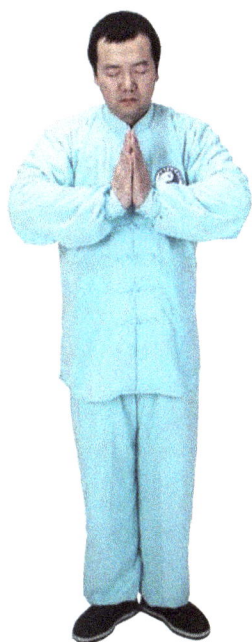

接前势，缓缓起立，两脚收回，仍脚尖着地，两掌不变。

Slowly stands up and take back the feet, still keeping the palms and touching the floor with the toes.

图6-4　Fig 6-4

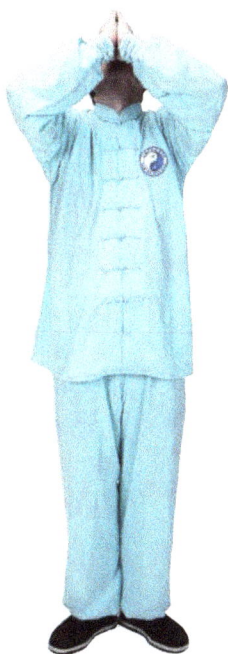

接前势，将脚跟慢慢放平立定，缓缓将头向后倒仰，朝天合掌，以仰面朝天为度。

Slowly put the heels down, make the head lean backward (with the face towards the sky) and close the palms.

图6-5　Fig 6-5

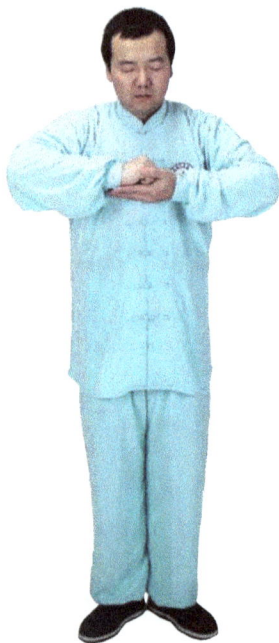

接前势，缓缓顺势回转、返回
第一势。

Slowly turn back and return to
movement # 1.

图6-6　Fig 6-6

第七势　九鬼拔马刀
Movement # 7　Nine Ghosts Drawing Swords

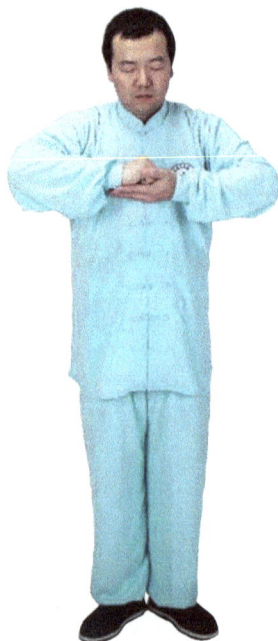

两足开立，脚跟并拢，两脚
尖成八字形，两臂自然下垂于体
侧；身胸挺直，两目平视，定心凝
神；然后两手缓缓上抬，两脚同
时缓缓立起，屈肘于胸前，合掌。

Stand upright with separated
feet, put the heels together, turn toes
of both feet outward and drop the
arms naturally to the sides. Keep the
body upright, look straight ahead
and cleanse the mind. Slowly lift
the hands and feet, flex the elbows
in front of the chest and close the
palms.

图7-1　Fig 7-1

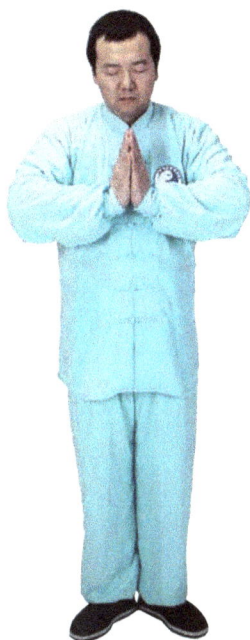

接前势，双手打开，回抱合掌，指尖齐于鼻尖。

Open the hands, then take back and close the palms, making the fingertips at the same level of the nasal tip.

图7-2　Fig 7-2

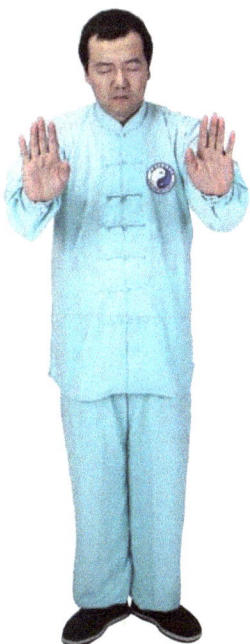

稍停一会，将手尽力向前推出，立掌，与肩齐，两掌底与两肩角相对。稍停一会，接着两掌回收、平肩，掌立。

Pause for a while and then make an effort to push forward. Keep the palms upright at the same level of the shoulders and let the soles facing to the humeral angles. Pause for a while, take back the palms, square the shoulder and keep the palms upright.

图7-3　Fig 7-3

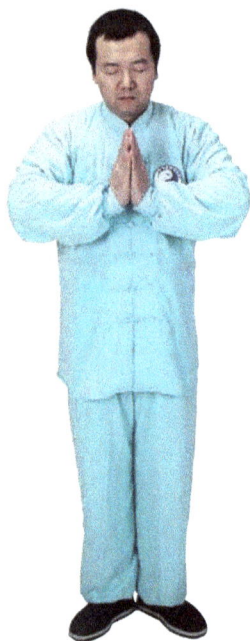

接前势,两掌回收,平肩,掌立。

Take back the palms, square the shoulder and make the palms upright.

图7-4　Fig 7-4

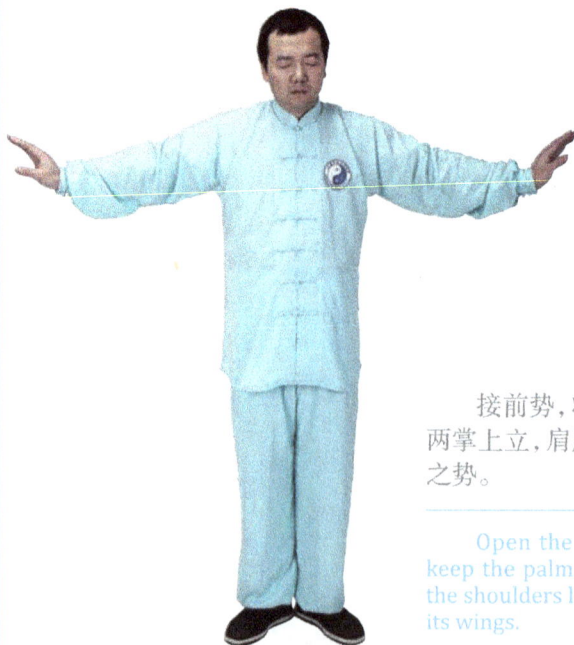

接前势,将两手向两侧撑开,两掌上立,肩膀平直,如飞鹰展翅之势。

Open the hands to both sides, keep the palms upright, and square the shoulders like an eagle spreading its wings.

图7-5　Fig 7-5

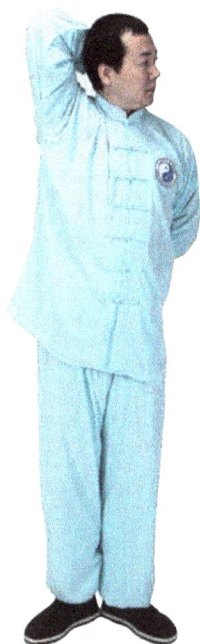

接上式，右拳变掌由腹侧缓
缓上抬，至上臂与耳平行时，拔
肩，屈肘，弯腰，扭项，使右掌心向
内，停于左侧面部，成抱头状；同
时左拳变掌，置于背后，尽力上
抬，定式后静立。

Turn the right fist into palm and
slowly lift from the ventral aspect
until the upper arm to the level of the
ear. Pull the shoulder, flex the elbow,
bend the waist and turn the neck.
Make the right palm inward, place
at the left side of the face and form a
head-holding position. Turn the left
fist into palm, place behind the back,
make an effort to lift the left palm and
stand still.

图7-6　Fig 7-6

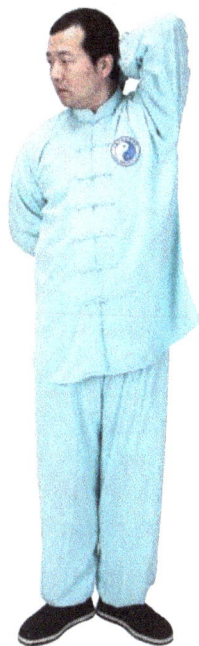

然后，左右手势互换，依上法
而行。停立30秒至10分钟，循序
渐进，量力而行。

Then perform the same procedure
in an opposite direction. Stay still from
30 seconds to 10 minutes according to
individualized body condition.

图7-7　Fig 7-7

［诀曰］侧首弯肱，抱顶及颈；自头收回，弗嫌力猛：左右相轮，身直气静。

[Tips] Flex the arm to move the head and neck, do not use strenuous exertion, perform on left and right side alternately, keep the body upright and breathe naturally.

［功效］柔软肢体，疏通经络，增长本力。

[Functions] This movement unblocks meridians, enables the limbs to be more flexible and increase physical strength.

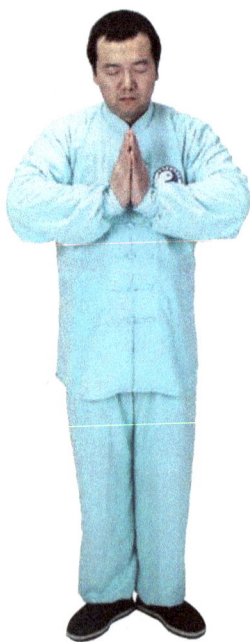

图7-8　Fig 7-8

接前势，双手先向两侧打开，接着慢慢回抱合掌，指尖齐于鼻尖。

Open the hands to both sides, slowly take back and close the palms and make the fingertips at the level of the nasal tip.

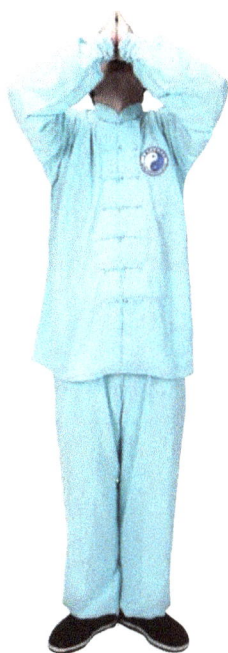

接前势，将脚跟慢慢放平立
定，缓缓将头向后倒仰，朝天合
掌，以仰面朝天为度。

Slowly put the heels down, make
the head lean backward (with the face
towards the sky) and close the palms.

图7-9　Fig 7-9

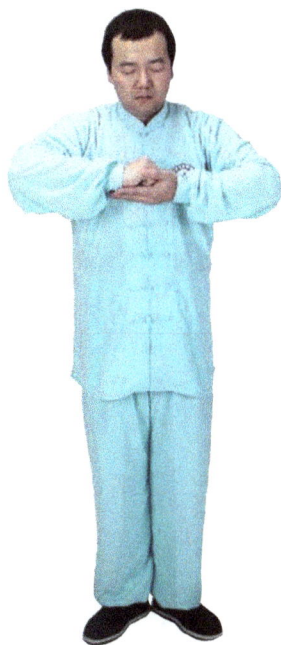

接前势，缓缓顺势回转，返回
第一势。

Slowly turn back and return to
movement # 1.

图7-10　Fig 7-10

第八势 三盘落地

Movement # 8　Three Plates Falling on the Floor

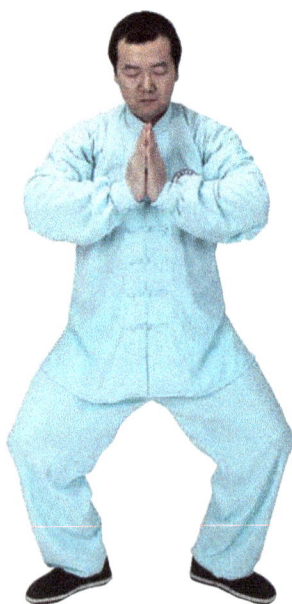

图8-1　Fig 8-1

将脚跟离地,下身如骑马势,两脚成外八字,大腿与小腿成90°,双手合掌于胸前,上身中正,下坐。

Lift the heels off the floor, make the lower body a horse riding posture and turn the toes of both feet outward, forming approximately 90° between the thigh and lower leg. Close the palms in front of the chest, and keep the upper body upright and lower body down.

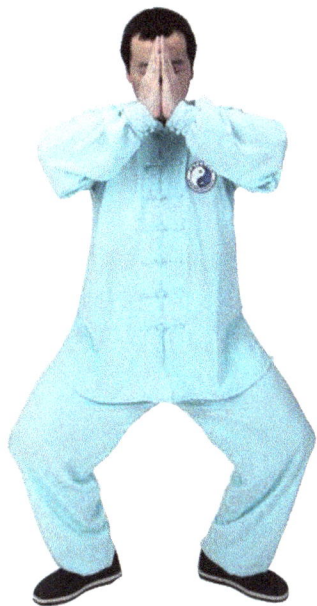

接前势，将合掌初放在神庭
上；次推上泥丸宫；然后由泥丸
向上尽力一撑，如在马上打恭状
(图8-2，图8-3)。

图8-2　Fig 8-2

Close the palms and place on
Shenting[1] (DU 24). Push the palms
up to Baihui[2] (DU 20) (*Ni Wan Gong*).
Then prop up the palms like bowing
with clasped hands on a horse. (Fig
8-2, Fig 8-3)

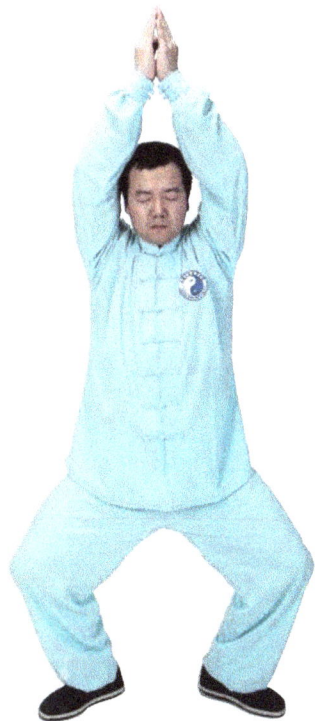

图8-3　Fig 8-3

1. An acupuncture point located on the head, .5 cun directly above the midpoint of the
anterior hairline.
2. An acupuncture point located at the midpoint of the line connecting the apexes of the two
auricles.

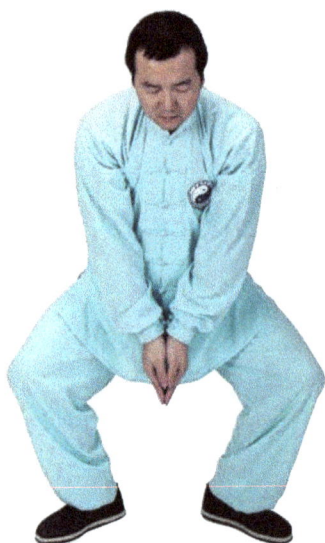

图8-4　Fig 8-4

接前势，合掌打恭至地，膀伸肱直、头正身直，向下一撑；然后起身还原。继续打恭，三上三下，其功乃全。

Close the palms, bow with clasped hands on the floor, extend the arms, keep the head and body upright, and prop down. Then stands up and continue to bow with clasped hands, 3 times of upward and 3 times of downward.

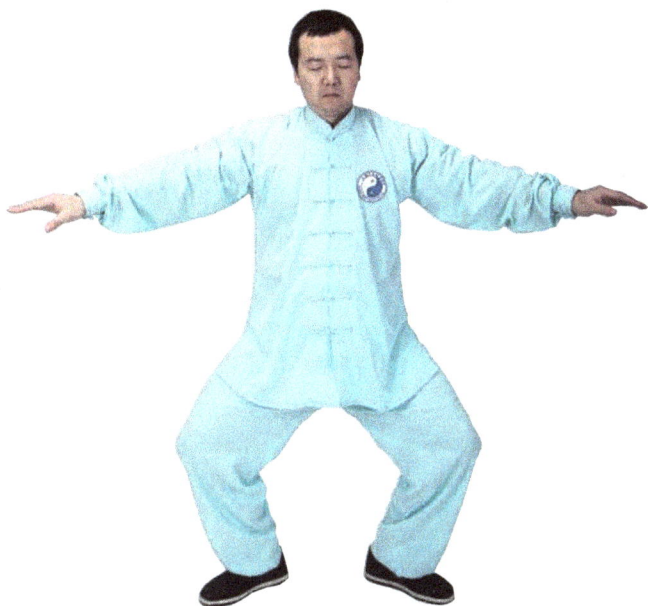

图8-5   Fig 8-5

接上式,两掌向两侧打开,两腿屈膝半蹲成马步,挺胸塌腰;同时左掌下落,右掌由背后移于身前,然后两臂向两侧成伞状展开并下按,掌心朝下。定式后调息,然后两掌反掌向上托,如拾重物;臂平胸时,两腿屈膝,两手反掌下按,重复马步式。上述动作反复做3次。前后停立30秒至10分钟,循序渐进,量力而行。

Open the palms to both sides, bend at the knees to form a horse stance, chest out, and relax the waist. Drop the left palm, shift the right palm from back to the front of the body and open the arms to both sides like an umbrella and press down with the palms downward. Breathe naturally, turn the palms and lift up as if carrying a heavy object. Extend the arms to the level of the chest, bend at the knees, turn the palms to press down and repeat the horse stance. Repeat 3 times and stay still from 30 seconds to 10 minutes according to individualized body condition.

[诀曰] 上腭坚撑舌,张眸意注牙;足开蹲似踞,手按猛如拿;两掌翻齐起,千斤重有加;瞪目兼闭口,起立足无斜。

[Tips] Touch the palate with the tongue, separate the feet to squat, press hard with the hands, turn the palms upward, and keep the mouth closed and eyes wide open.

[功效] 调理脏腑,疏通经络,增长体能。

[Functions] This movement regulates zang-fu organs, unblocks meridians and increases the physical strength.

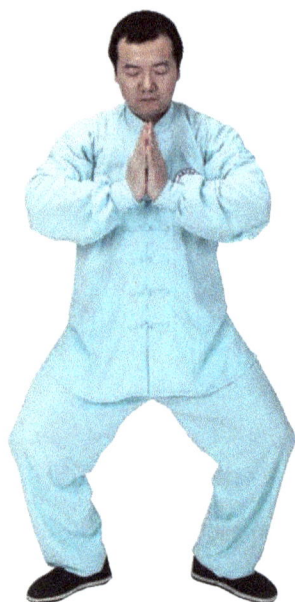

接前势，缓缓将双手收回，到胸前合掌，返回第一势。

Take back and close the hands in front of the chest, return to movement #1.

图8-6　Fig 8-6

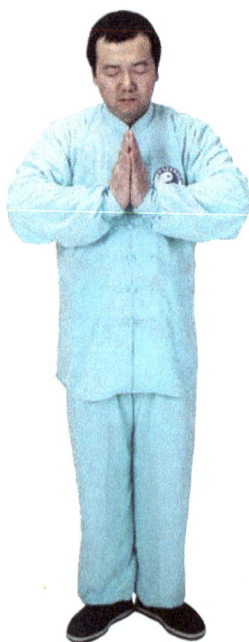

接前势，缓缓起立，两脚收回，仍脚尖着地，两掌不变。

Slowly stands up and take back the feet, still keeping the palms and touching the floor with the toes.

图8-7　Fig 8-7

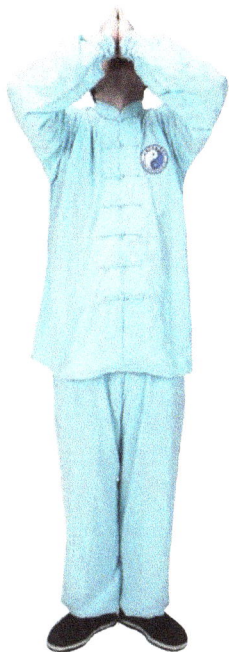

接前势,将脚跟慢慢放平立定,缓缓将头向后倒仰,朝天合掌,以仰面朝天为度。

Slowly put the heels down, make the head lean backward (with the face towards the sky) and close the palms.

图8-8　Fig 8-8

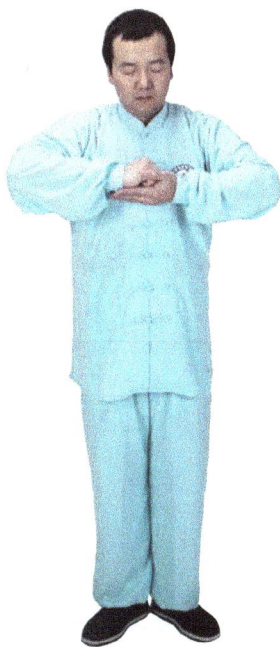

接前势,缓缓顺势回转,返回第一势。

Slowly turn back and return to movement # 1.

图8-9　Fig 8-9

第九势　青龙探爪

Movement # 9　Black Dragon Displaying Its Claws

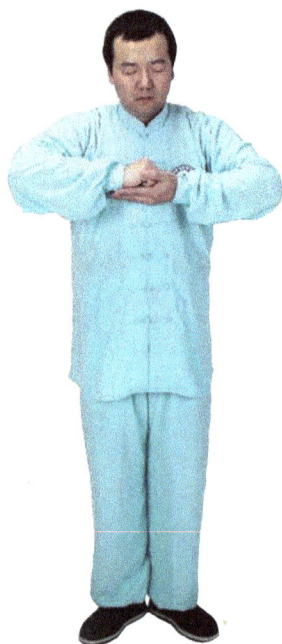

图9-1　Fig 9-1

　　两足开立,脚跟并拢,两脚尖成八字形,两臂自然下垂于体侧;身胸挺直,两目平视,定心凝神;然后两手缓缓上抬,两脚同时缓缓立起,屈肘于胸前,合掌。

Stand upright with separated feet, put the heels together, turn toes of both feet outward and drop the arms naturally to the sides. Keep the body upright, look straight ahead and cleanse the mind. Slowly lift the hands and feet, flex the elbows in front of the chest and close the palms.

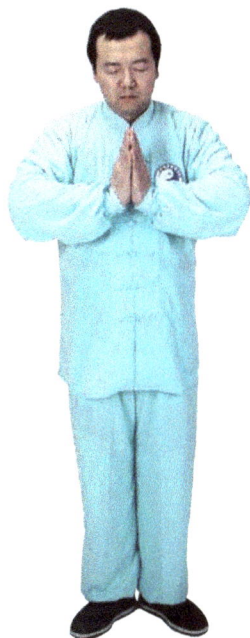

图9-2　Fig 9-2

接前势，双手打开，回抱合掌，指尖齐于鼻尖。稍停一会，将手尽力向前推出，立掌，与肩齐，两掌底与两肩角相对。稍停一会，接着两掌回收，平肩，掌立(图9-2、图9-3)。

Open the hands, then take back and close the palms, making the fingertips at the same level of the nasal tip. Pause for a while and then make an effort to push forward. Keep the palms upright at the same level of the shoulders and let the soles facing to the humeral angles. Pause for a while, take back the palms, square the shoulder and keep the palms upright. (Fig 9-2, Fig 9-3)

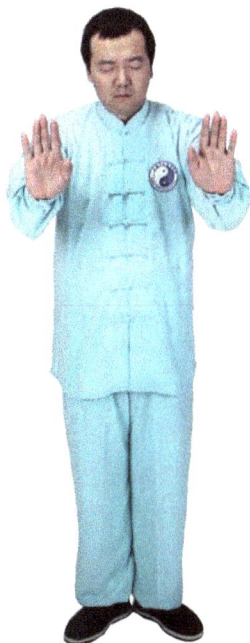

图9-3　Fig 9-3

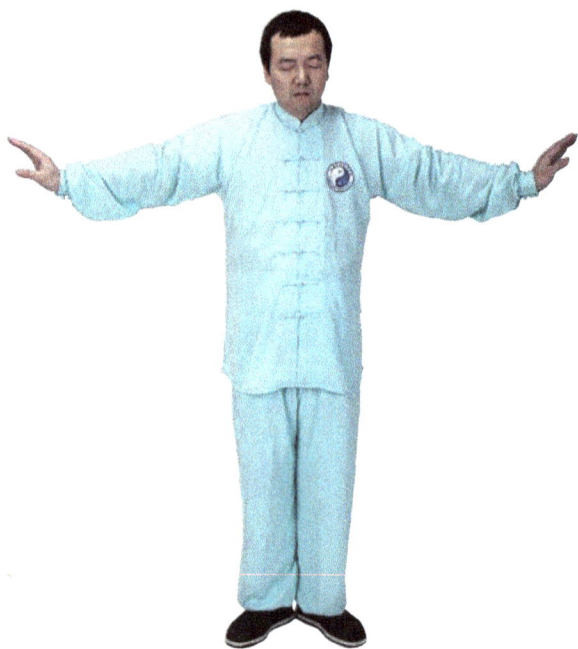

图9-4   Fig 9-4

接前势,将两手向两侧撑开,两掌上立,肩膀平直,如飞鹰展翅之势,两掌缓缓撑开。

Open the hands to both sides, keep the palms upright, and square the shoulders like an eagle spreading its wings. Then slowly prop up the palms.

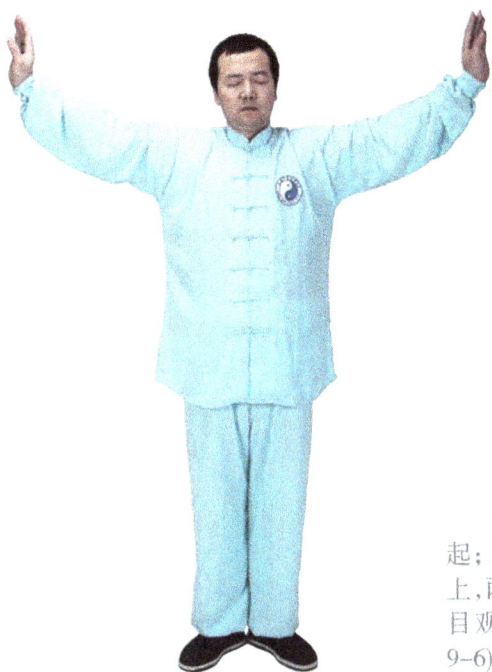

图9-5　Fig 9-5

两脚开立，足尖着地，足跟提起；双手上举高过头顶，掌心向上，两中指相对；沉肩曲肘，仰头，目观掌背，鼻息调匀(图9-5、图9-6)。

Separate the feet with toes touching the floor and lift the heels off the floor. Lift the hands above the top of the head, with the palms upward and two middle fingers facing each other. Drop the shoulders, flex the elbows, focus the eyes on the dorsa of the palms and breathe naturally with the nose. (Fig 9-5, Fig 9-6)

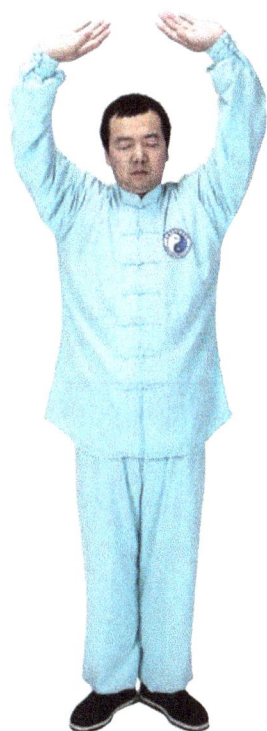

图9-6　Fig 9-6

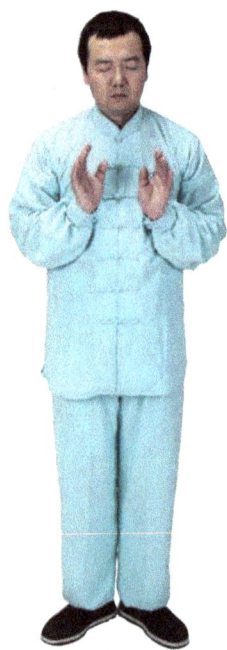

图9-7　Fig 9-7

　　接前势，将两掌顺左右势直下，向外直立至两肩角；膀肱曲折，两腋挟紧。

　　Drop the palms to left and right humeral angles, with the palms upright. Flex the arms and tighten the armpits.

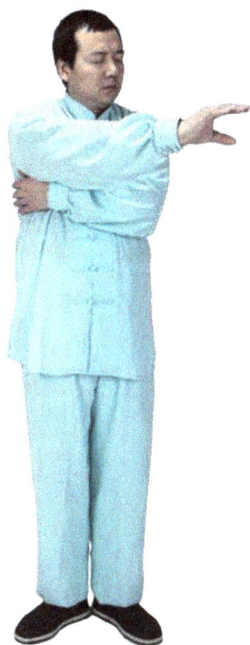

图9-8　Fig 9-8

接上式,收左脚落右脚内侧半步,使两腿成并排步;身胸挺直,两目平视,左掌经胸前变拳,抱于腰侧,拳心向上,右掌绕胸前变"五花屈爪"形,向左侧伸探。然后左右手势互换,依上法而行。左右式反复做九遍。停立30秒至10分钟,循序渐进、量力而行(图9-8、图9-9)。

Take back the left foot half a step to the medial side of the right foot like the position of 'standing at attention'. Keep the body upright and look straight ahead. Turn the left palm into a fist in front of the chest and place the fist on the left side of the waist. Turn the right palm into a claw hand in front of the chest to extend towards the left. Then perform the same procedure with the left hand and repeat 9 times. Stay still from 30 seconds to 10 minutes according to individualized body condition. (Fig 9-8, Fig 9-9)

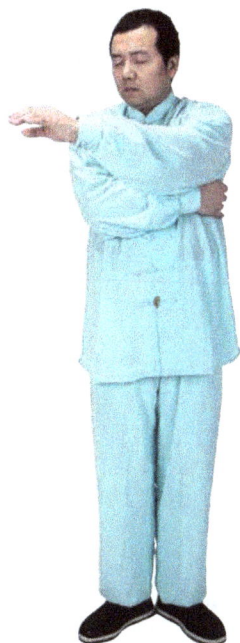

图9-9　Fig 9-9

　　［诀曰］青龙探爪，左从右出；修士效之，掌气平实；力周肩背，围收过膝；两目平注，息调心谧。

　　[Tips] Display the left claws from the right side (vice versa), push palms with the force from the shoulder and back, look straight ahead and breathe naturally with the nose.

　　［功效］调理肢体，疏通经络，增长脚力。

　　[Functions] This movement regulates the limbs, unblocks meridians and increases the strength of the feet.

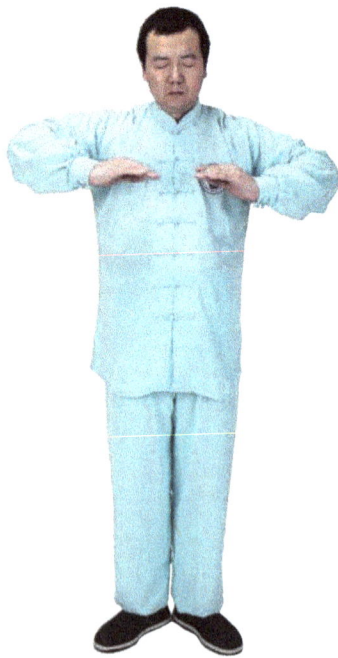

图9-10　Fig 9-10

　　接前势，与右同。势毕，将两手收回至颈项。接前势，将掌心向下，掌背向上，指尖相对；膀与肩直；左右一撑。

　　Take back the hands to the neck and nape area. Make the centers of the palms downward and fingertips face each other. Extend the arms to the level of the shoulders and prop up to both sides.

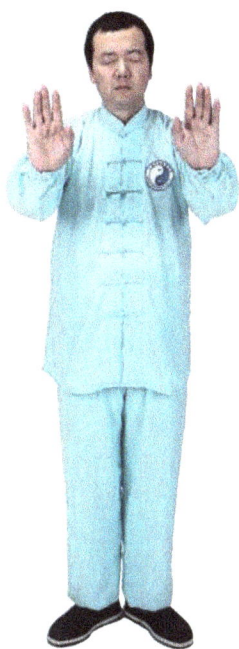

接前势，将手尽力向前推出，立掌，与肩齐，两掌底与两肩角相对。

Make an effort to push the hands forward, keep the palms upright at the level of the shoulders and let the bottom of the palms opposite to the humeral angles.

图9-11　Fig 9-11

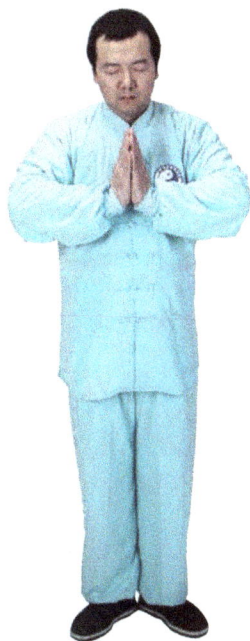

接前势，双手打开，回抱合掌，指尖齐于鼻尖。

Open the hands, then take back and close the palms, making the fingertips at the level of the nasal tip.

图9-12　Fig 9-12

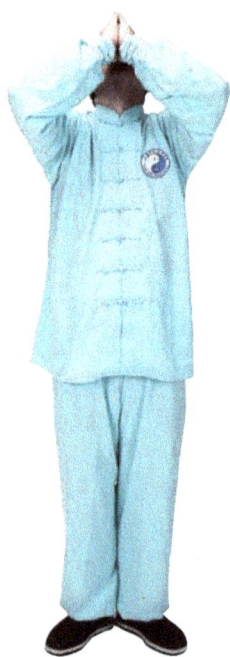

接前势，将脚跟慢慢放平立定，缓缓将头向后倒仰、朝天合掌，以仰面朝天为度。

Slowly put the heels down, make the head lean backward (with the face towards the sky) and close the palms.

图9-13　Fig 9-13

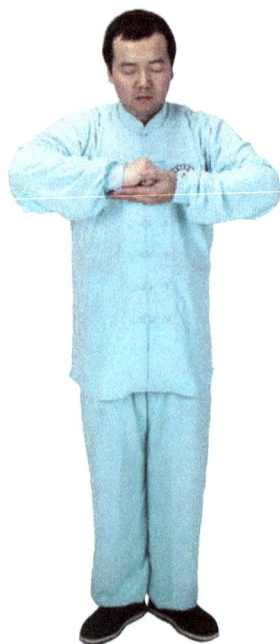

接前势，缓缓顺势回转，返回第一势。

Slowly turn back and return to movement # 1.

图9-14　Fig 9-14

第十势 卧虎扑食

Movement # 10　Hungry Tiger Springing on Its Prey

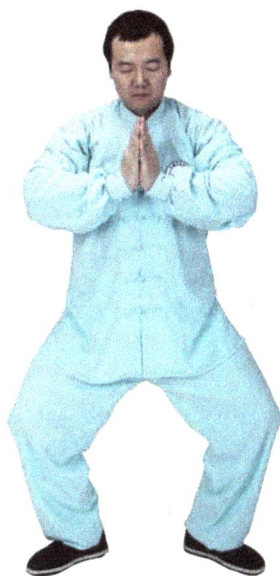

图10-1　Fig 10-1

　　将脚跟离地,下身如骑马势,两脚成外八字,大腿与小腿成90°,双手合掌于胸前,上身中正,下坐。

Lift the heels off the floor, make the lower body a horse riding posture and turn the toes of both feet outward, forming approximately 90° between the thigh and lower leg. Close the palms in front of the chest, and keep the upper body upright and lower body down.

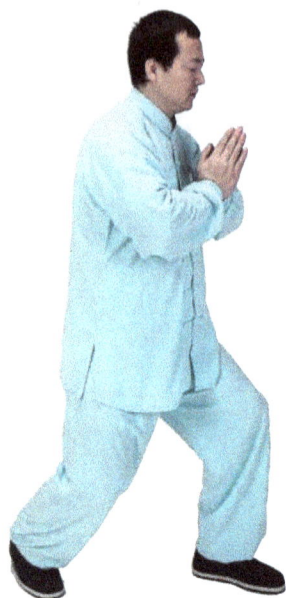

图10-2　Fig 10-2

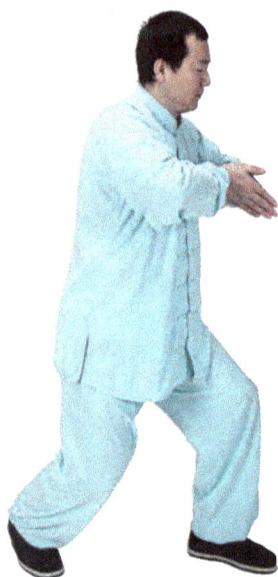

图10-3　Fig 10-3

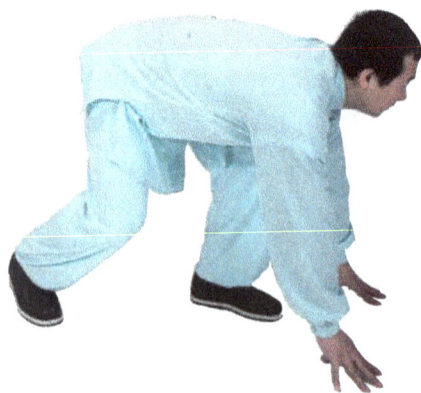

图10-4　Fig 10-4

接上式，两掌在胸前不变；身体向左转，左腿屈，右腿弯直，脚跟提起，成左弓步；同时俯身、拔肩、塌腰、昂头，两掌指着地。定式后静立（图10-2、图10-3、图10-4）。

Further to the last movement (with the palms in front of the chest), turn the body left, flex the left leg, extend the right leg, lift the right heel off the floor and form a left bow step. Bend the body, pull the shoulder, relax the waist, raise the head and touch the floor with the palms and ten fingers. Stay still for a while. (Fig 10-2, Fig 10-3, Fig 10-4)

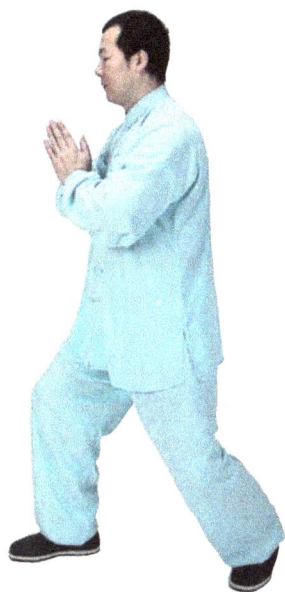

图10-5　Fig 10-5

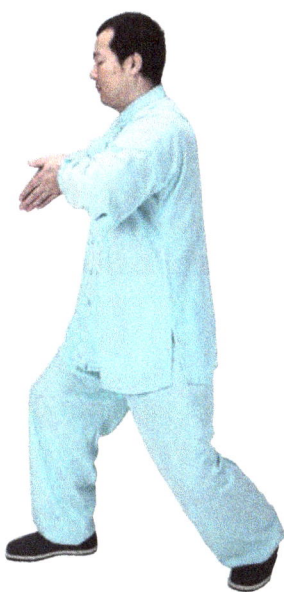

图10-6　Fig 10-6

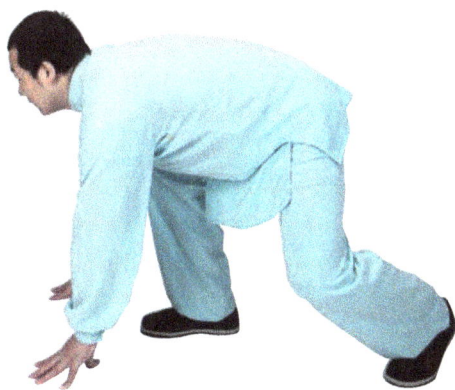

图10-7　Fig 10-7

　　然后缓缓起身，两脚碾地，体向右转，成右弓步，左脚跟提起，同时俯身、拔脊、塌腰、昂头，两掌指着地。定式后静立。停立30秒至10分钟，循序渐进，量力而行（图10-5、图10-6、图10-7）。

Then slowly stand up and touch the floor with the feet. Turn the body right and form a right bow step by lifting the left heel off the floor. Bend the body, pull the shoulder, relax the waist, raise the head and touch the floor with the palms and ten fingers. Stay still from 30 seconds to 10 minutes according to individualized body condition. (Fig 10-5, Fig 10-6, Fig 10-7)

［诀曰］两足分蹲身似倾，屈伸左右腿相更；昂头胸作探前势，偃背腰还似砥平；鼻息调元均出入，指尖著地赖支撑；降龙伏虎神仙事，学得真形也卫生。

[Tips] Flex the left and right leg alternately, raise the head to prey, breathe naturally with the nose, and focus the mental concentration on fingers.

［功效］柔韧肢体，理气，疏通脊柱，增强体质。

[Functions] This movement regulates qi, benefits the spine, makes the limbs more flexible and increases the body constitution.

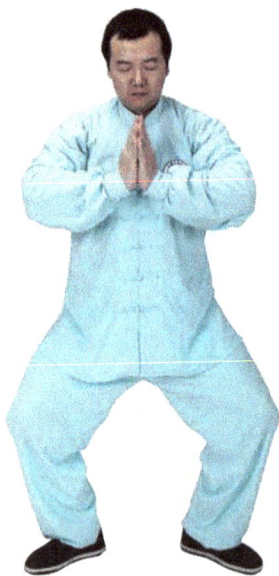

图10-8   Fig 10-8

接前势。缓缓起身，还原。脚跟离地，下身如骑马势，两脚成外八字，大腿与小腿成90°，双手合掌于胸前，上身中正，下坐。

Slowly stands up, lift the heels off the floor, make the lower body a horse riding posture and turn the toes of both feet outward, forming approximately 90° between the thigh and lower leg. Close the palms in front of the chest, and keep the upper body upright and lower body down.

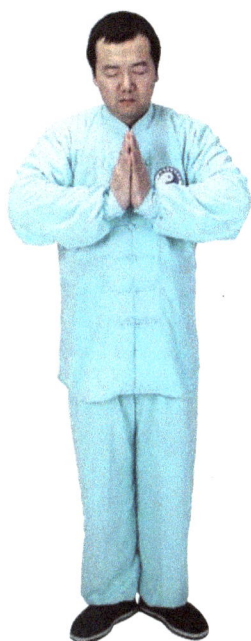

接前势，缓缓起身，双手合掌
于胸前，指尖齐于鼻尖。

Slowly stands up, close the
hands in front of the chest and make
the fingertips at the level of the nasal
tip.

图10-9　Fig 10-9

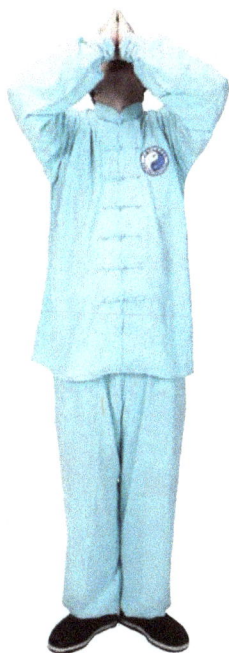

接前势，将脚跟慢慢放平立
定，缓缓将头向后倒仰，朝天合
掌，以仰面朝天为度。

Slowly put the heels down, make
the head lean backward (with the face
towards the sky) and close the palms.

图10-10　Fig 10-10

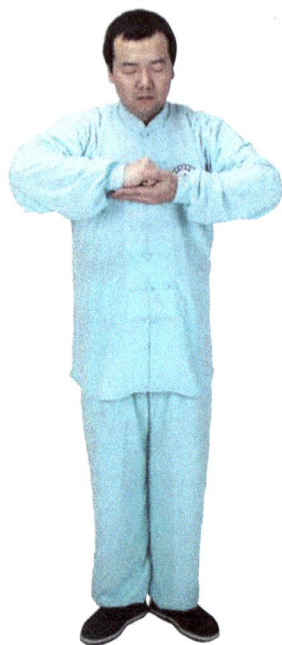

接前势，缓缓顺势回转，返回第一势。

Slowly turn back and return to movement # 1.

图10-11　Fig 10-11

第十一势　打躬
Movement # 11　Bowing Down in Salutation

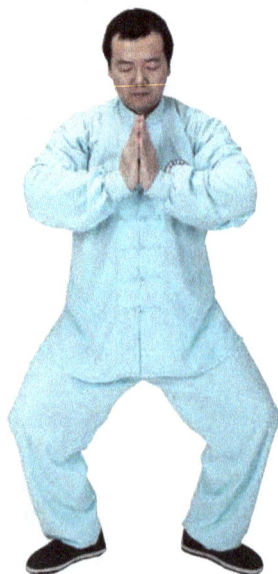

将脚跟离地，下身如骑马势，两脚成外八字，大腿与小腿成90°，双手合掌于胸前，上身中正，下坐。

Lift the heels off the floor, make the lower body a horse riding posture and turn the toes of both feet outward, forming approximately 90° between the thigh and lower leg. Close the palms in front of the chest, and keep the upper body upright and lower body down.

图11-1　Fig 11-1

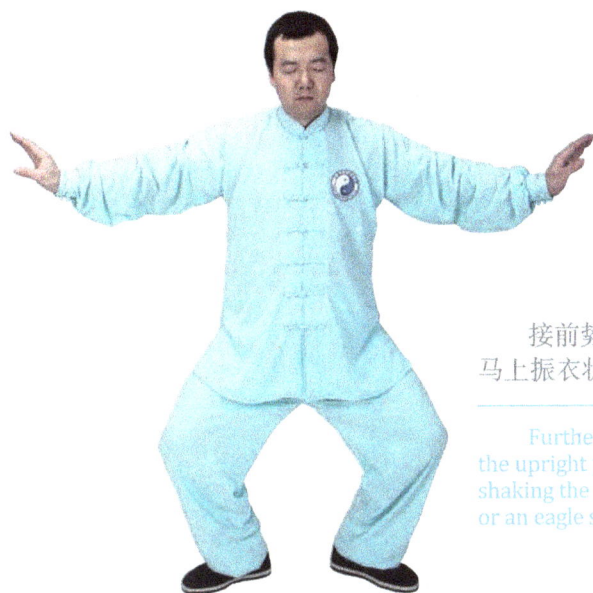

接前势，向左右立掌撑开，如
马上振衣状，又像飞鹰展翅。

Further to movement # 1, open
the upright palms to left and right like
shaking the dust off clothes on a horse
or an eagle spreading its wings.

图11-2 Fig 11-2

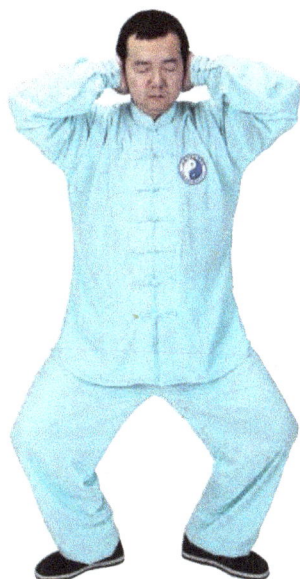

接前势，将两掌头按伏两耳，
两手中三指紧按天柱，正身平视，
一志凝神。

Use the palms to press the ears
and use the index, middle and ring
fingers to press Tianzhu[1](BL 10). Keep
the body upright, look straight ahead
and concentrate the mind.

图11-3 Fig 11-3

1. An acupuncture point located on the lateral aspect of the trapezius muscle, 1.3 cun
lateral to Yamen (DU 15) [1.5 cun directly above the midpoint of the posterior hairline,
below the 1st cervical vertebra].

接上式，缓缓起身；向前慢慢俯身、躬腰、垂脊、挺膝，头部探于胯下；同时两臂随身向前屈肘，环附于项后，两掌心掩塞两耳，然后两掌夹抱后脑。定式后静立。停立30秒至10分钟，循序渐进，量力而行。

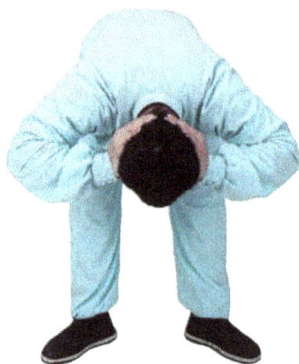

Slowly stand up, bend forward, bow at the waist, stretch the spine, extend the knees and put the head down below the crotch. Flex the elbows forward and move to the back of the neck. Cover the ears with the palms and then use the palms to hold the occiput. Stay still from 30 seconds to 10 minutes according to individualized body condition.

图11-4　Fig 11-4

［诀曰］两手齐持脑，垂腰至膝间；头惟探胯下，口更齿牙关；掩耳聪教塞，调元气自闲；舌尖还抵腭，力在肘双弯。

[Tips] Hold the occiput with both hands, bow at the waist, put the head down below the crotch, cover the ears with the palms, use the tongue tip to touch the palate and exert force from the elbows.

［功效］调理脊柱，理气，疏通背部经络，增长脚力。

[Functions] This movement benefits the spine, unblocks meridians on the back and increases the strength of the feet.

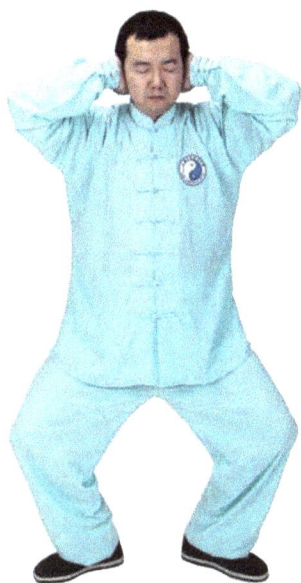

接前势，缓缓起身，将两掌头按伏两耳，两手中三指紧按天柱，正身平视，一志凝神。

Slowly stand up, use the palms to press the ears and use the index, middle and ring fingers to press Tianzhu (BL 10). Keep the body upright, look straight ahead and concentrate the mind.

图11-5　Fig 11-5

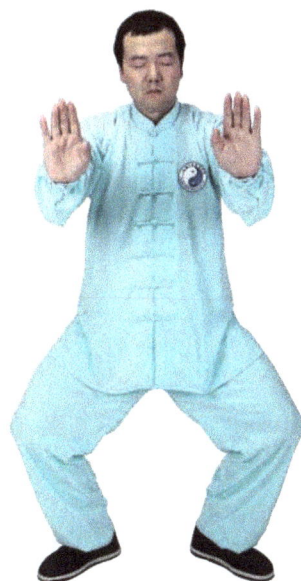

接前势，两掌顺势向前推出，余法同前。

Push the palms forward.

图11-6　Fig 11-6

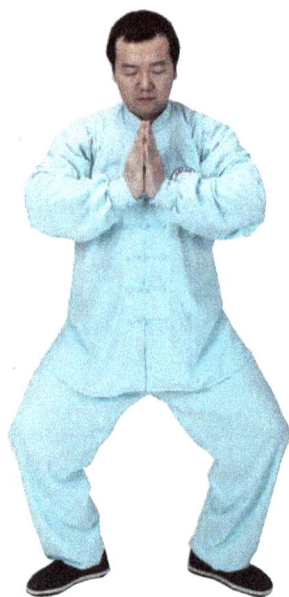

接前势，将两掌缓缓收回至胸前，脚跟离地，下身如骑马势，两脚成外八字，大腿与小腿成90°，双手合掌于胸前，上身中正，下坐。

Take back the palms to the front of the chest, lift the heels off the floor, make the lower body a horse riding posture and turn the toes of both feet outward, forming approximately 90° between the thigh and lower leg. Close the palms in front of the chest, and keep the upper body upright and lower body down.

图11-7　Fig 11-7

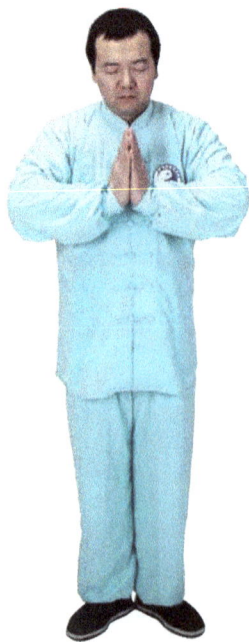

接前势，缓缓起身，双手合掌于胸前，指尖齐于鼻尖。

Slowly stands up, close the palms in front of the chest and make the fingertips at the level of the nasal tip.

图11-8　Fig 11-8

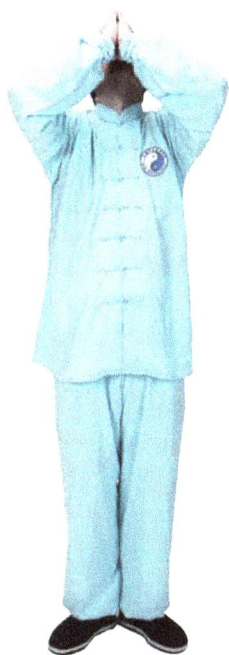

接前势，将脚跟慢慢放平立定，缓缓将头向后倒仰，朝天合掌，以仰面朝天为度。

Slowly put the heels down, make the head lean backward (with the face towards the sky) and close the palms.

图11-9　Fig 11-9

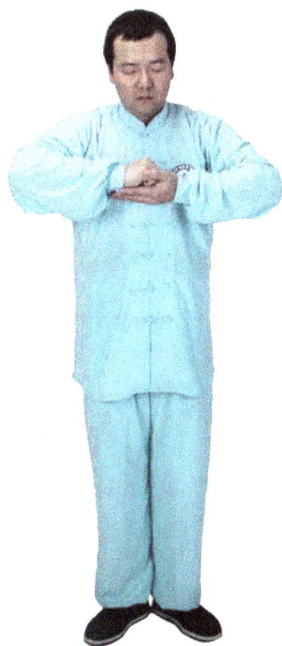

接前势，缓缓顺势回转，返回第一势。

Slowly turn back and return to movement # 1.

图11-10　Fig 11-10

第十二势　掉尾

Movement # 12　Swinging the Tail

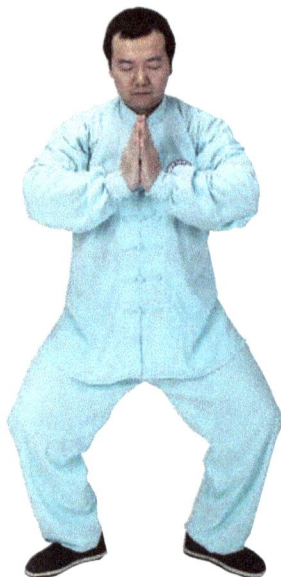

此势将脚跟离地，下身如骑马势，两脚成外八字，大腿与小腿成90°，双手合掌于胸前，上身中正，下坐。

Lift the heels off the floor, make the lower body a horse riding posture and turn the toes of both feet outward, forming approximately 90° between the thigh and lower leg. Close the palms in front of the chest, and keep the upper body upright and lower body down.

图12-1　Fig 12-1

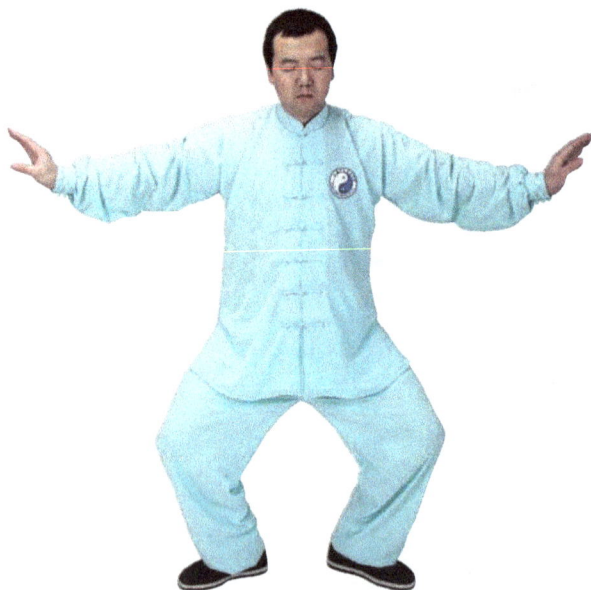

图12-2　Fig 12-2

接前势，向左右立掌撑开，如马上振衣状，又像飞鹰展翅。

Further to movement # 1, open the upright palms to left and right like shaking the dust off clothes on a horse or an eagle spreading its wings.

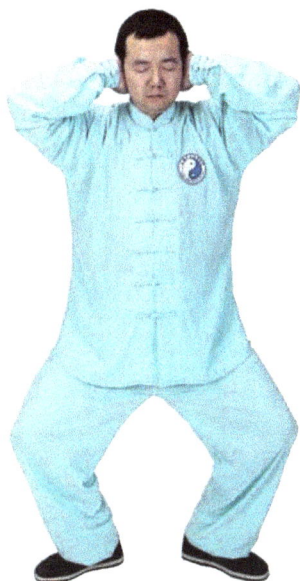

接前势，将两掌头按伏两耳，两手中三指紧按天柱，正身平视，一志凝神。

Use the palms to press the ears and use the index, middle and ring fingers to press Tianzhu (BL 10). Keep the body upright, look straight ahead and concentrate the mind.

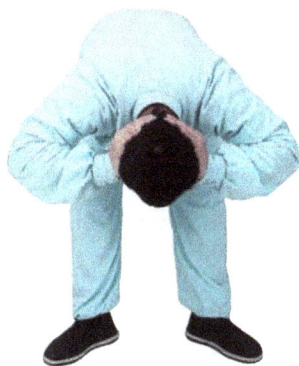

图12-3　Fig 12-3

接上式，缓缓起身；向前慢慢俯身、躬腰、垂脊、挺膝，头部探于胯下；同时两臂随身向前屈肘，环附于项后，两掌心掩塞两耳，然后两掌夹抱后脑。

Slowly stand up, bend forward, bow at the waist, stretch the spine, extend the knees and put the head down below the crotch. Flex the elbows forward and move to the back of the neck. Cover the ears with the palms and then use the palms to hold the occiput.

图12-4　Fig 12-4

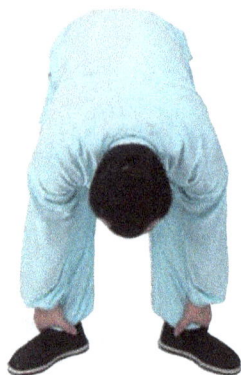

接前势，将两掌放松，由后颈项挨身顺下至两足边，手搬脚踝对立，膝关节与踝关节尽量挺直，俯首凝神。

Release the palms and drop from the nape to both sides of the feet, use the hands to grasp the ankles, make an effort to extend the knee and ankle joints and bow the head with a concentrated mind.

图12-5　Fig 12-5

接上式，提膝，十趾尖着地；两臂顺两腿下垂，两手指贴住脚背，轻轻抓住脚趾；同时仰头，两目圆睁，视鼻尖，凝神谧志。定式后足跟落地，然后再提起足跟，重复3次，再伸膀挺肘一次，共提跟顿地21次，伸膀7次，功毕起立，收式归原。停立30秒至10分钟，循序渐进，量力而行。

Lift the knees and touch the floor with ten toes. Drop the arms along the legs and use the fingers to touch the dorsa of the feet and grasp the toes. Lean the head backward, make the eyes wide open, focus the eyes on the nasal tip and concentrate the mind. Then touch the floor with the heels and re-lift the heels off the floor. Repeat 3 times and then extend the arms and elbows. There are a total of 21 times of lifting the heels off the floor and touching the floor and 7 times of extending the arms. Return to the neutral position and stay still from 30 seconds to 10 minutes according to individualized body condition.

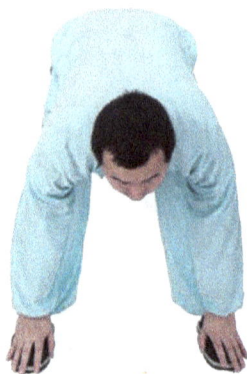

图12-6　Fig 12-6

［诀曰］膝直膀伸，推手自地；瞪目昂头，凝神一志；起而顿足，二十一次；左右伸肱，以七为志；更作坐功，盘膝垂眦；口注于心，息调于鼻；定静乃起，厥功维备。

[Tips] Extend the knees and arms, keep the eyes wide open, cleanse the mind, repeat 21 times of lifting the heels off the floor and touching the floor and 7 times of extending the left and right arm and regulate breathing through the nose.

［功效］疏通脊柱经络，调整肢体，增长体力。

[Functions] This movement unblocks Du meridian, strengthens the four limbs and increases physical strength.

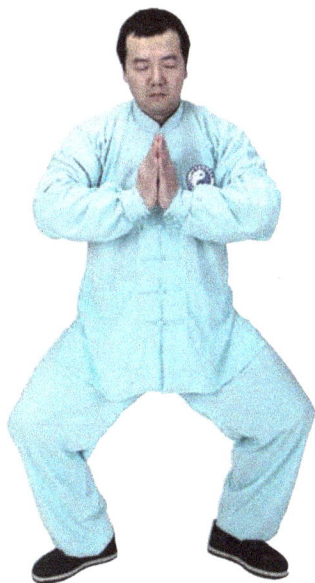

接前势，缓缓起身，身随头起，足尖点地，合掌定气于胸前。

Slowly lift the head and body, touch the floor with the toes and close the palms in front of the chest.

图12-7　Fig 12-7

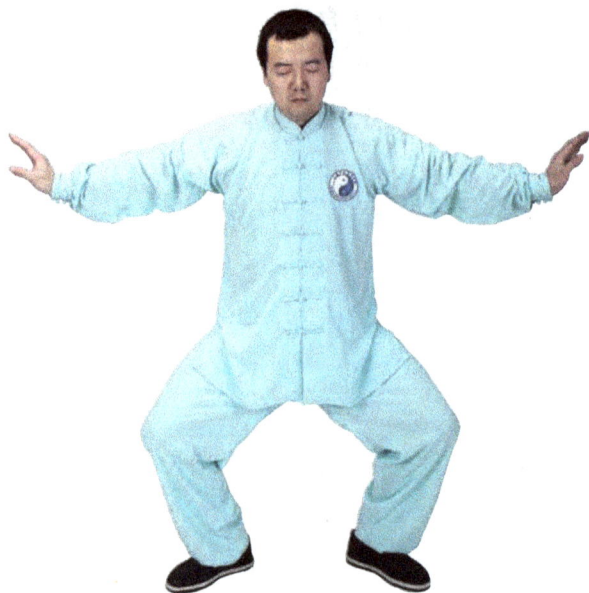

图12-8　Fig 12-8

接前势,将两手向左右撑开,舒畅血脉,宽胸理气,立掌,与肩对齐。

Open the hands to left and right to soothe the chest, regulate qi and circulate blood. Make the palm upright to the level of the shoulders.

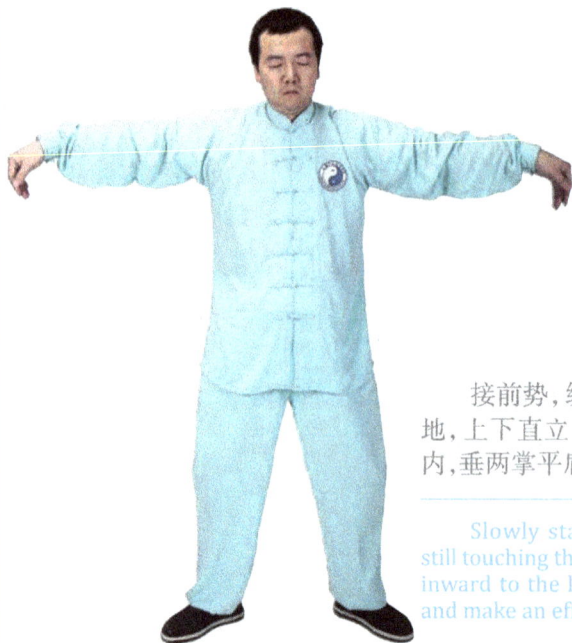

接前势,缓缓起身,仍足尖点地,上下直立,掌背向外,掌心向内,垂两掌平肩,尽力上提。

Slowly stand up with the toes still touching the floor, turn the palms inward to the level of the shoulders and make an effort to lift the arms.

图12-9　Fig 12-9

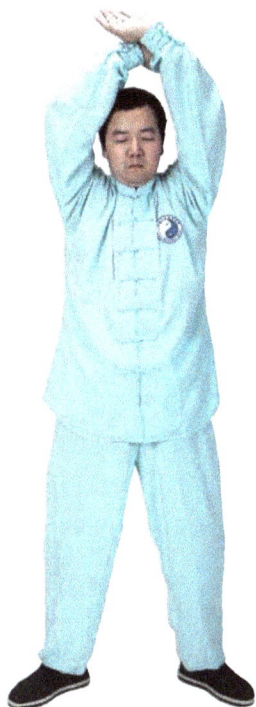

接前势，将两掌心逆翻至顶，交叉，顺势着力向左右拨开，以膀伸肱直为度，而上下身直，足仍离地，恍如踏云拨雾之状。

Turn the palms over the top of the head, cross the palms and open up to both sides until the arms are extended. Keep the body upright with the heels off the floor, like walking on clouds and clearing the fog.

图12-10　Fig 12-10

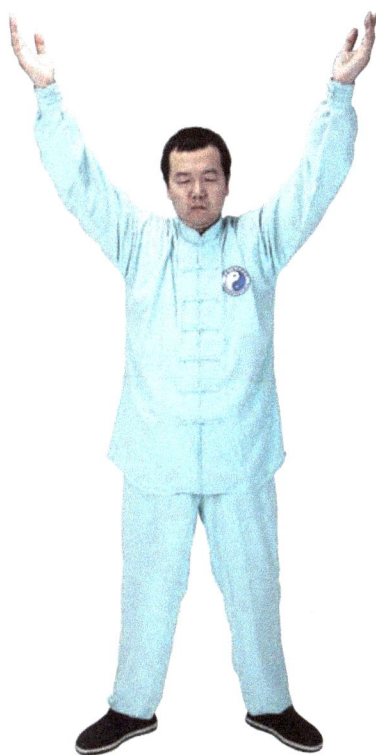

接前势，仍足尖点地，上下身直，将两掌心翻转，排左右朝天，尽力往上下一撑，上托下镇。

With toes touching the floor, keep the body upright, turn the palms upward and make an effort to prop up.

图12-11　Fig 12-11

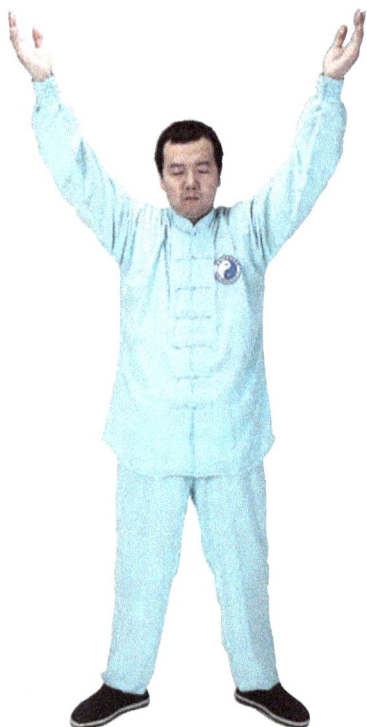

接前势，将两手向左右排开，阳掌向外，阴掌向内，使左手与右脚对，右手与左脚对，然后四肢一撑。

Open the hands to left and right, with yang palm outward and yin palm inward. Make the left hand facing the right foot and the right hand facing the left foot. Then extend the four limbs.

图12-12　Fig 12-12

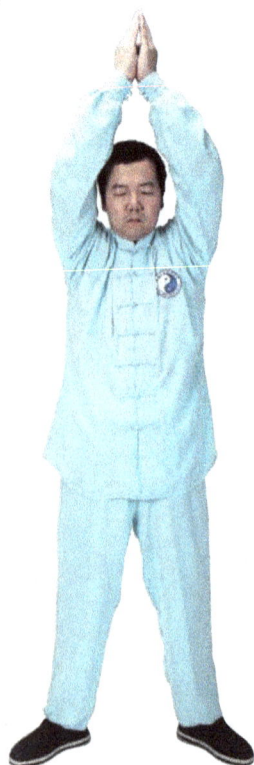

接前势，将两手收至头顶，合掌直伸，悬吊如钟。

Return the hands over the top of the head, close and straighten the palms like a hanging bell.

图12-13　Fig 12-13

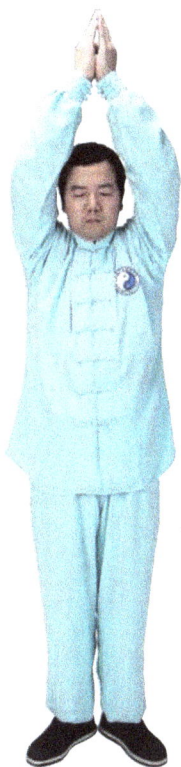

接前势，将两脚收回，足根相
碰，仍起脚离地，上下一撑，直立
如松。

Take back the feet and put the
heels together. Lift the heels off the
floor to prop up and stand upright
like a pine tree.

图12-14　Fig 12-14

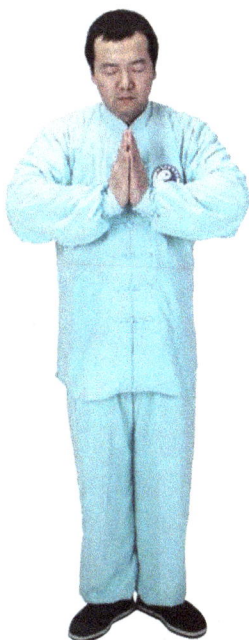

接前势，将手掌缓缓收回，合
掌于胸前，指尖齐于鼻尖。平肩。

Slowly take back the palms and
close them in front of the chest. Place
the fingertips at the level of the nasal
tip and square the shoulders.

图12-15　Fig 12-15

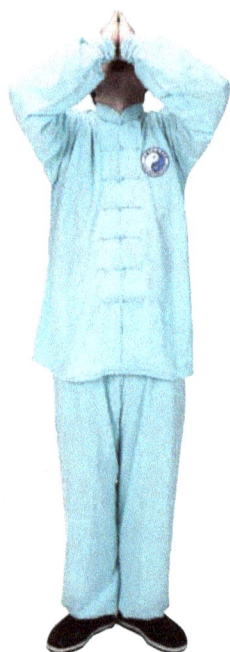

接前势,将脚跟慢慢放平立定,缓缓将头向后倒仰,朝天合掌,以仰面朝天为度。

Slowly put the heels down, make the head lean backward (with the face towards the sky) and close the palms.

图12-16   Fig 12-16

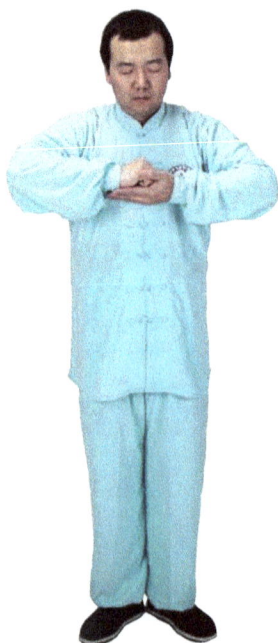

接前势,缓缓顺势回转,返回第一势。

Slowly turn back and return to movement # 1.

图12-17   Fig 12-17

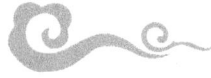

易 筋 经 ● *Yi Jin Jing* (Sinew-Transformation Classic)

Application

应用

易筋经是一种传统的导引方法,使人的精神、形体和气息有效地结合起来。经过循序渐进、持之以恒地锻炼,从而使五脏六腑及全身经脉得到充分的调理,进而达到保健强身,防病治病,抵御早衰,延年益寿的目的。

As a traditional Dao Yin exercise, *Yi Jin Jing* coordinates mental concentration, physical exercise and breathing. Persistent step-by-step exercise can benefit zang-fu organs and meridians, promote health, delay aging and achieve longevity.

强身健体
Strengthen the body

对于发育中的青少年,是行之有效的健身术。对虚弱的体质会大为改善,能使人神清气明,通身舒畅,可改善骨骼的结构,使之体健身强,气力渐增,可以有效地改善人体健康,许多疾病都会在练功中不药而愈。

Yi Jin Jing is beneficial for adolescents with a weak constitution. It can cleanse the mind, improve skeletal structure, increase physical strength and thus promote health. Many diseases can spontaneously recover after exercise of *Yi Jin Jing*.

体悟人生，净化心灵
Purify the mind

在不断的练功体悟中，反省自身，改变自己，完善自己。使自己不离正道，保持中庸，在不偏不倚，坚持正念中不断的净化自己的心灵，树立正确的道德观、世界观、人生观。使心身变得更健康，使生活更美好，让自己的心灵更自由。陶渊明云："既自以心为形役，奚惆怅而独悲？悟已往之不谏，知来者之可追。实迷途其未远，觉今是而昨非。"

During persistent exercise of *Yi Jin Jing*, one can reflect and then change or improve oneself. Over time, one can stay on the right track, do everything in moderation, use positive thinking to cleanse the mind and establish correct moral value and view of life and the world. 'Tao Yuan-ming[1] once said, 'I realize that the past is gone, but I can certainly rectify what is to come. I have not actually strayed too far from the path. I have awakened to today's rights and yesterday's wrongs.'

延缓衰老
Delay aging

随着年龄的增长，中年以后，身体功能逐渐衰退。到了老年，主要表现为肾虚肾亏、肌肉萎缩、腿脚不灵、动作迟缓，而易筋经能有效延缓这些衰老症状。通过脊柱锻炼，使脊椎伸拔，腰背松软灵活，脊髓通畅，同时也可整复脊柱的轻微变形，起到舒筋活血的作用。使任督二脉流通，强身固精，骨、髓、脑三者均得到充分滋养。血气旺盛，精气充满，则可不断地补益脑髓，使人

1. A Chinese poet during the Eastern Jin dynasty (317—420), particularly regarded as a Fields and Gardens poetry poet.

充满活力，头脑灵活、身轻体健。

The body function declines with age. People in old age often present with kidney deficiency, muscular atrophy, leg inflexibility and slow movements. *Yi Jin Jing* can delay these senile symptoms. Exercise of the spine can stretch the vertebrae, soften the low back, circulation qi and blood circulation along the Du meridian and adjust slightly deformed spine. Furthermore, exercise of *Yi Jin Jing* can unblock Ren and Du meridians, supplement essence to nurture the bone, marrow and brain and enable one to be lively, agile and energetic.

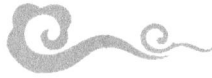

易　筋　经　·　*Yi Jin Jing* (Sinew-Transformation Classic)

The Meridian Charts

经络图

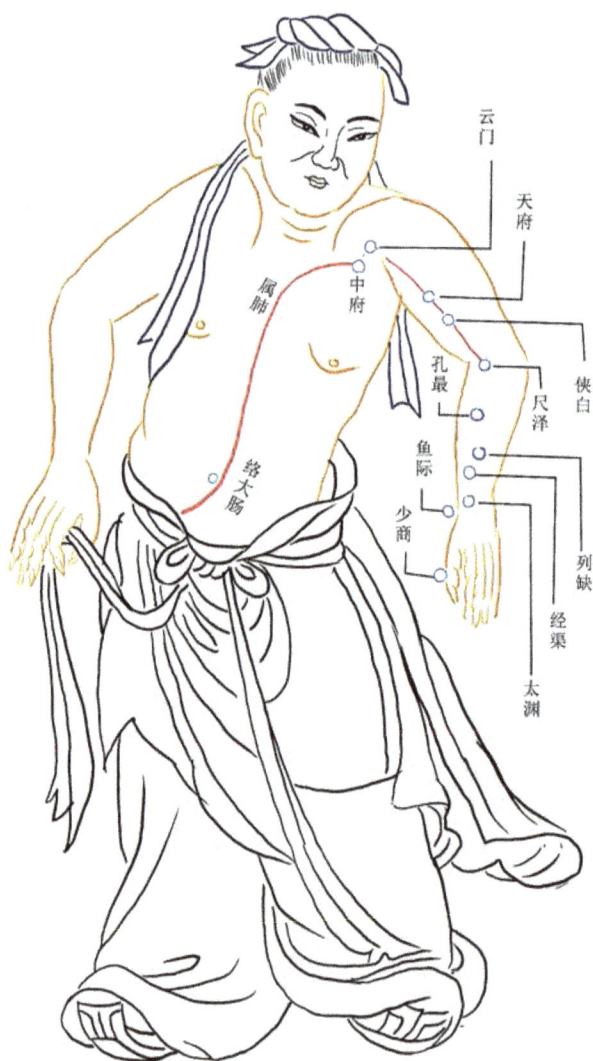

云门
天府
侠白
尺泽
列缺
经渠
太渊
少商
鱼际
孔最
中府
属肺
络大肠

手太阴肺经

Lung Meridian of Hand-Taiyin

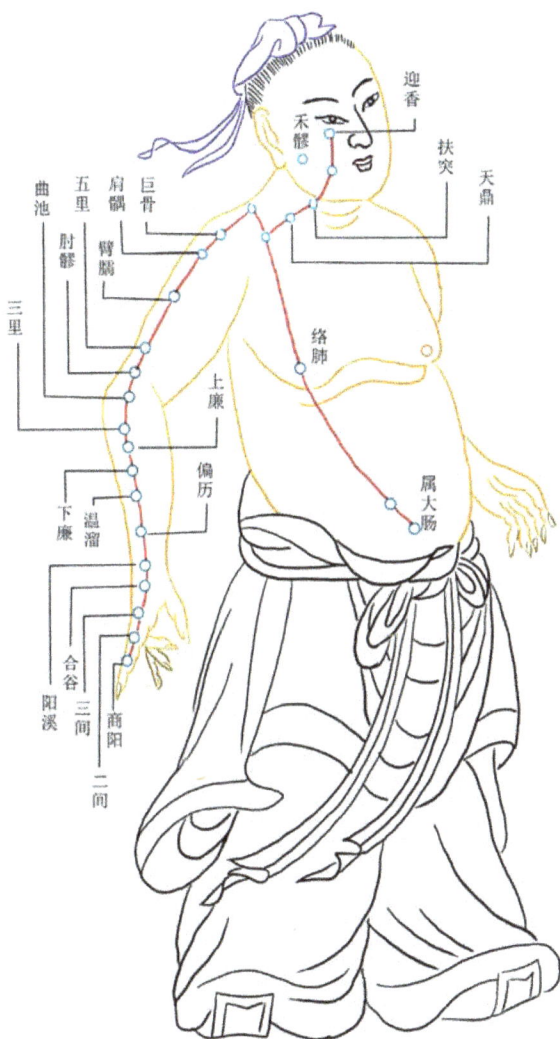

迎香
禾髎
扶突
天鼎
曲池
五里
肩髃
巨骨
臂臑
肘髎
三里
络肺
上廉
偏历
属大肠
下廉
温溜
合谷
三间
商阳
二间
阳溪

手阳明大肠经

Large Intestine Meridian of Hand-Yangming

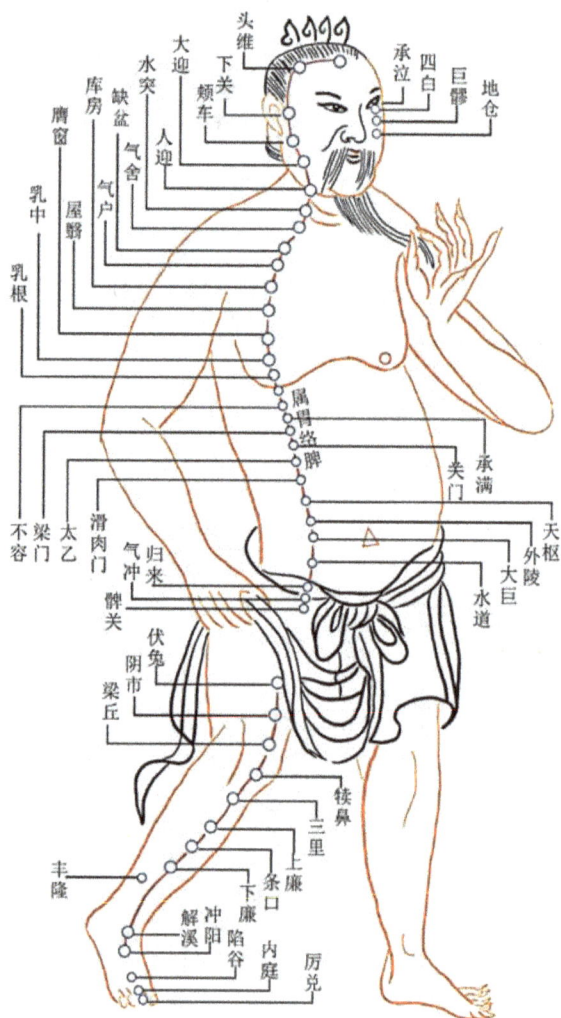

足阳明胃经

Stomach Meridian of Foot-Yangming

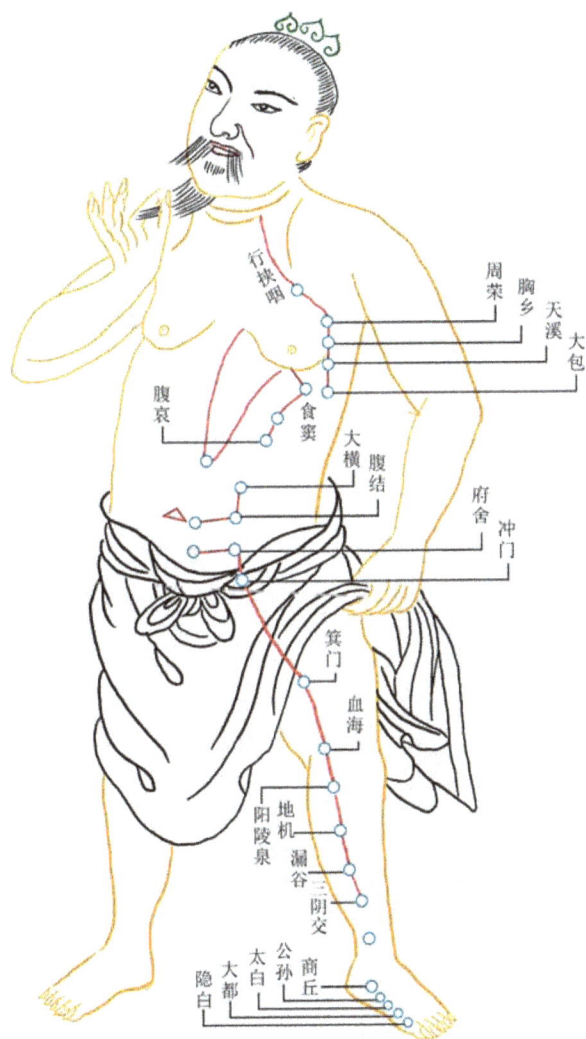

足太阴脾经

Spleen Meridian of Foot-Taiyin

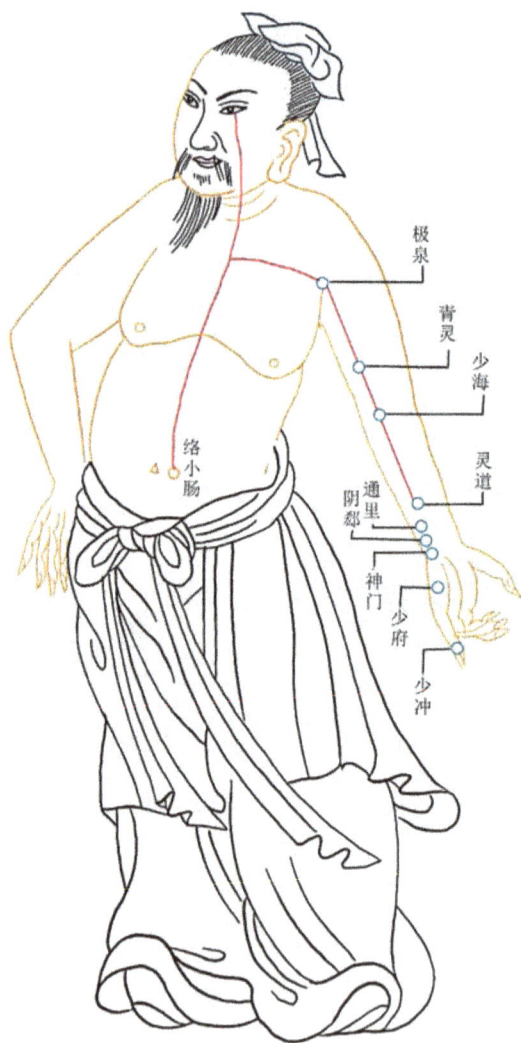

极泉

青灵

少海

灵道

通里

阴郄

神门

少府

少冲

络小肠

手少阴心经

Heart Meridian of Hand-Shaoyin

听宫
颧髎
天容
天窗
中俞
曲垣
秉风
肩贞
肩外俞
小海

膈俞
天宗
支正
养老
阳谷
腕骨
后溪
前谷
少泽

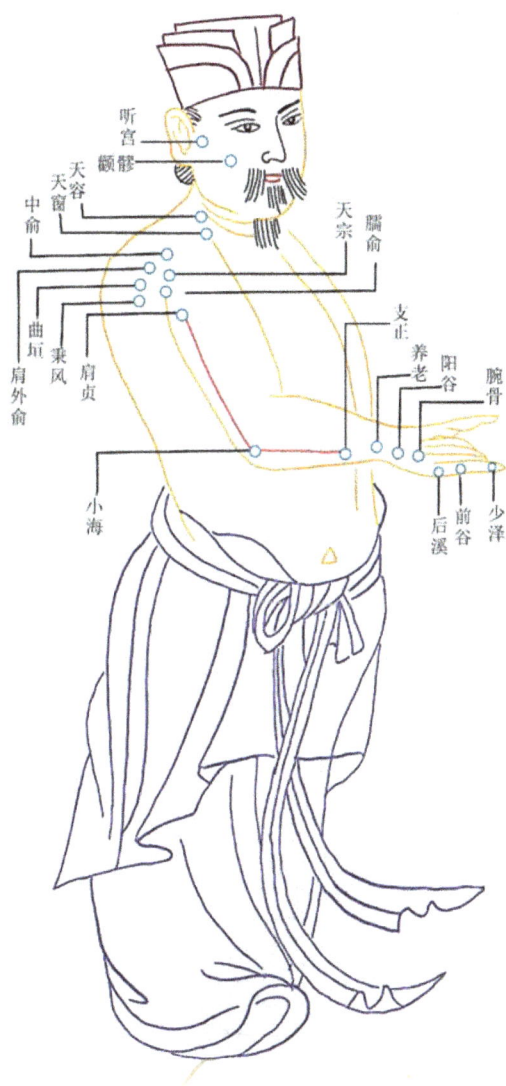

手太阳小肠经

Small Intestine Meridian of Hand-Taiyang

承光 五处 曲差 攒竹 睛明
附分
意舍 魄户 譩譆 神堂
膏肓
魂门 膈关 膈门 阳纲
肓门 志室 胃仓
腹肓
秩边
委阳 浮郄
承筋 承山 络飞阳 跗阳

通天 络却 玉枕
天柱 风门 大抒 肺俞 厥阴俞 心俞 膈腧
肝俞 胆俞
脾俞 胃俞 三焦俞 肾俞
大肠俞 小肠俞 膀胱俞 中膂俞 白环俞 会阳
承扶
殷门
合阳 委中
昆仑 仆参 申脉 金门 京骨 束骨 通谷 至阴

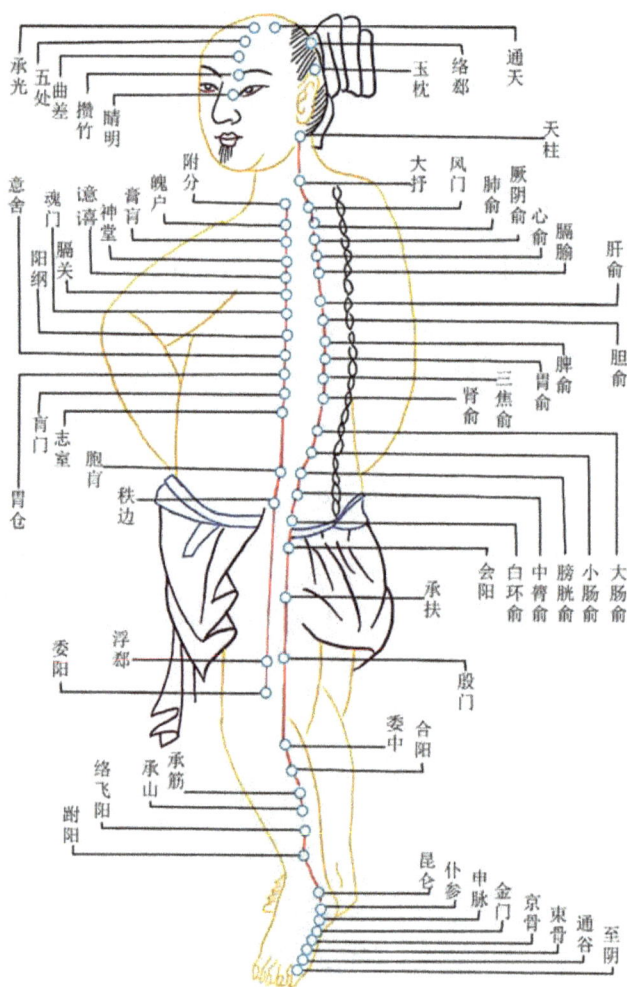

足太阳膀胱经

Bladder Meridian of Foot-Taiyang

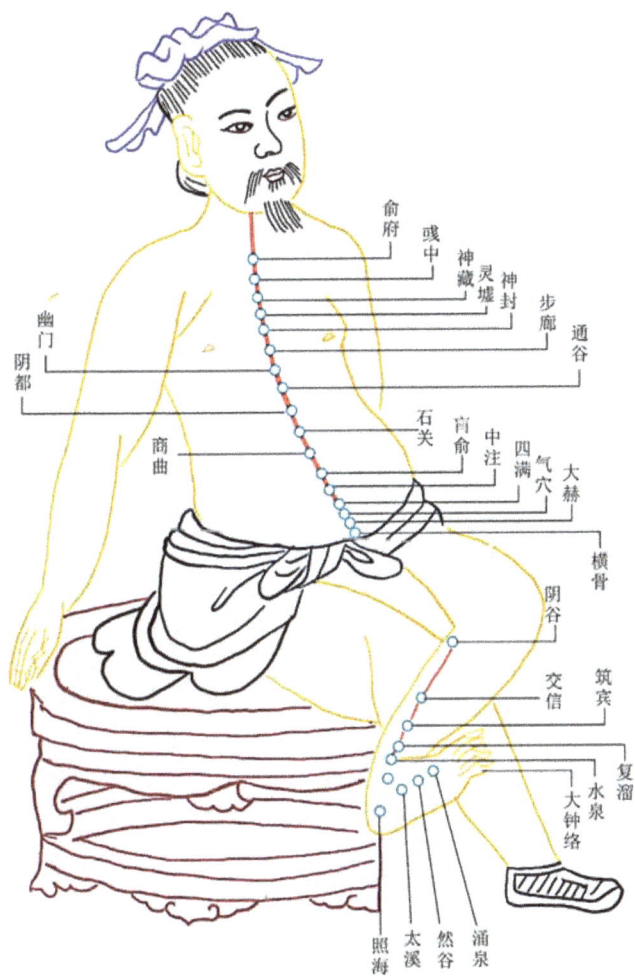

俞府
彧中
神藏　灵墟　神封
步廊
通谷
幽门
阴都
石关
肓俞　中注
商曲
四满
气穴
大赫
横骨
阴谷
交信　筑宾
复溜
水泉
大钟络
照海　太溪　然谷　涌泉

足少阴肾经

Kidney Meridian of Foot-Shaoyin

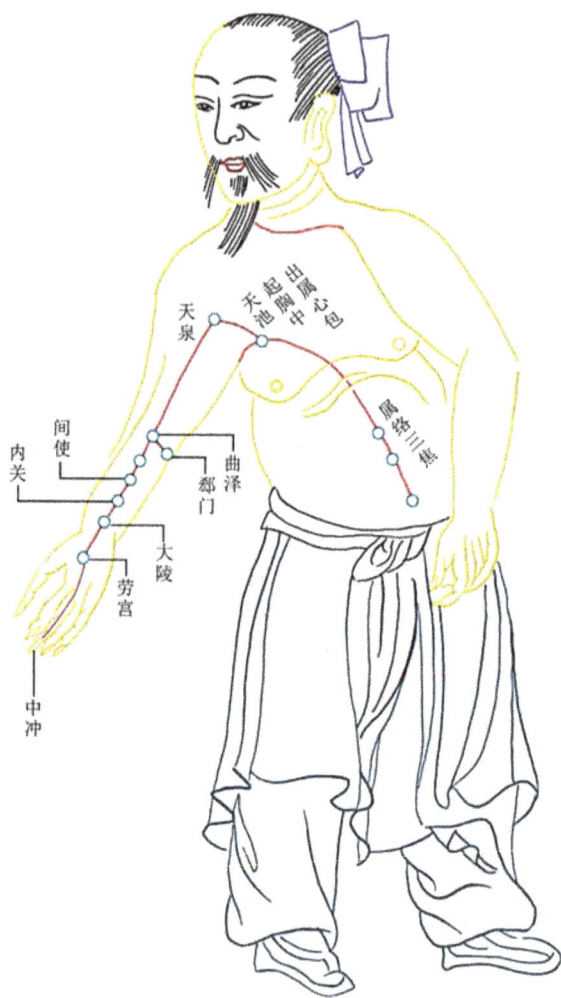

手厥阴心包经

Pericardium Meridian of Hand-Jueyin

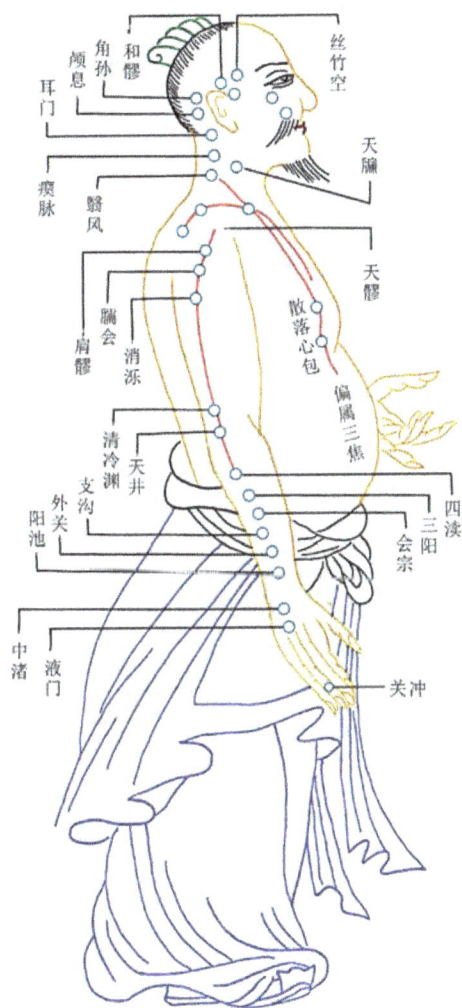

丝竹空
和髎
角孙
颅息
耳门
瘈脉
翳风
天牖
天髎
散落心包
臑会
肩髎
消泺
偏属三焦
清冷渊
天井
支沟
外关
阳池
四渎
三阳
会宗
中渚
液门
关冲

手少阳三焦经

Triple Energizer Meridian of Hand-Shaoyang

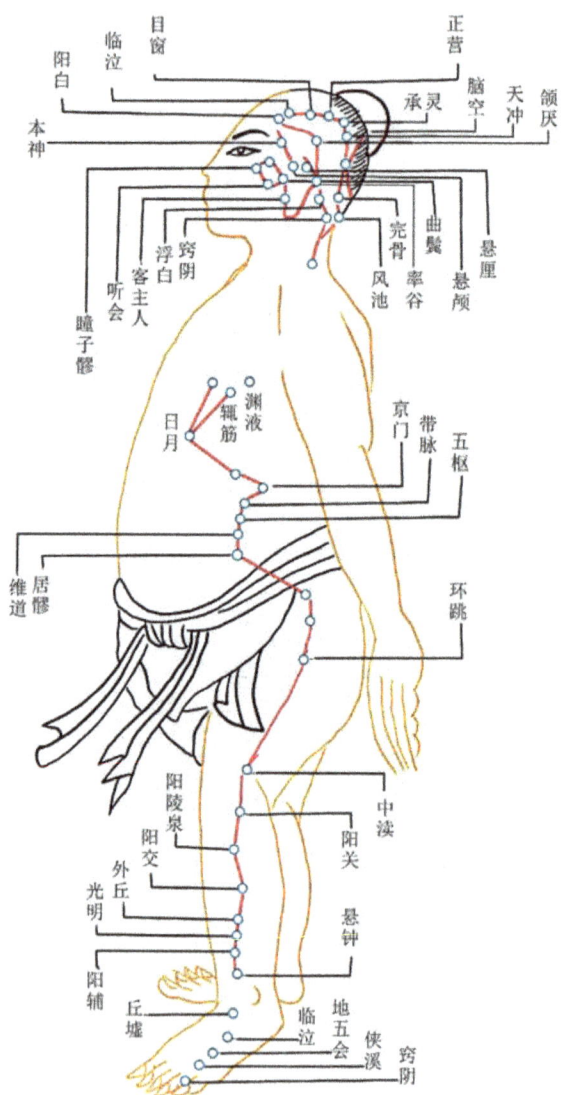

足少阳胆经

Gallbladder Meridian of Foot-Shaoyang

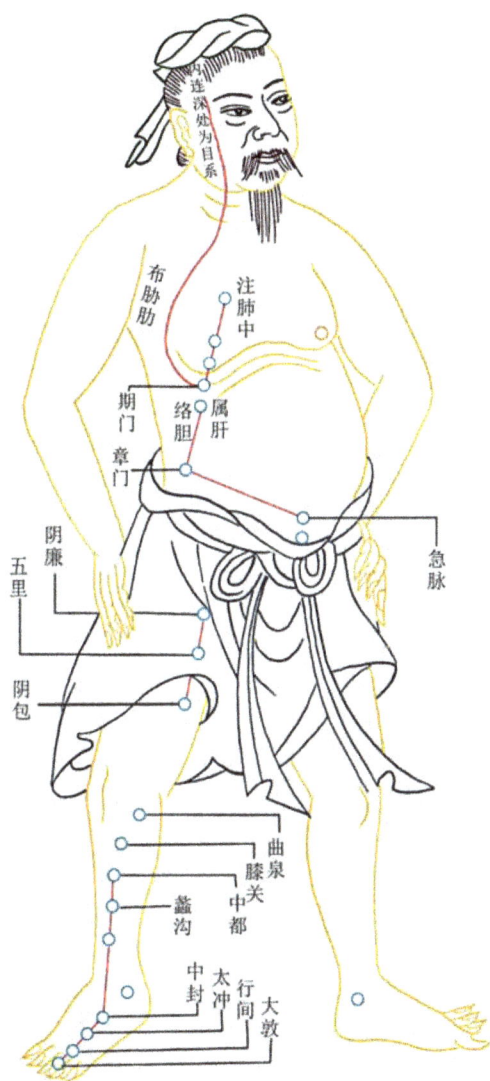

足厥阴肝经

Liver Meridian of Foot-Jueyin

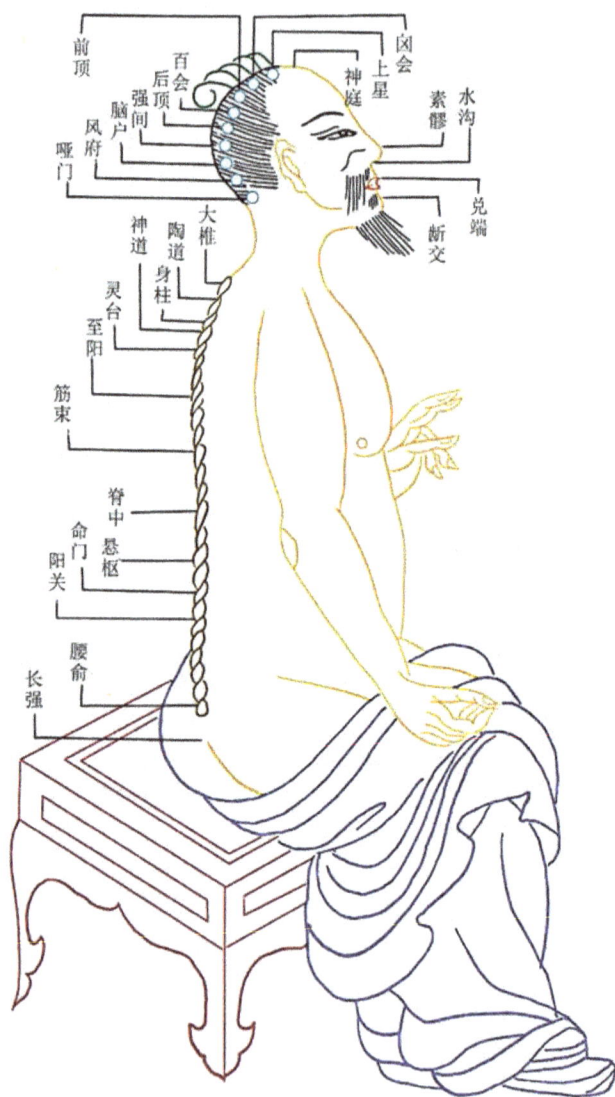

前顶
百会
后顶
强间
脑户
风府
哑门
神道
大椎
陶道
身柱
灵台
至阳
筋束
脊中
命门
阳关
腰俞
长强

囟会
上星
神庭
水沟
素髎
兑端
断交

督脉

Governor Vessel (Du)

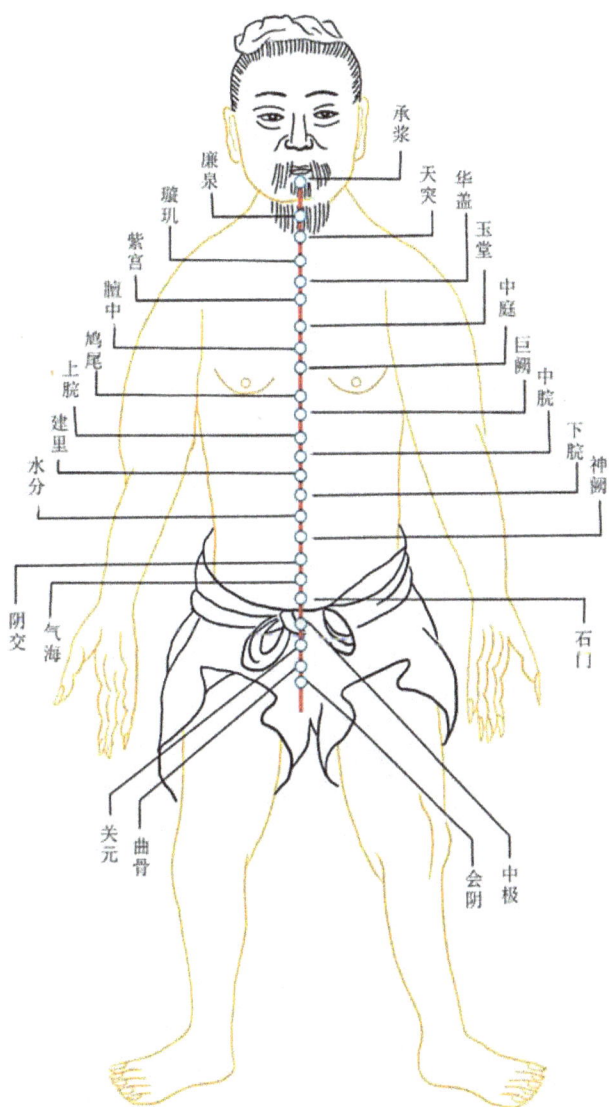

承浆
廉泉
璇玑
紫宫
膻中
鸠尾
上脘
建里
水分
阴交
气海
关元
曲骨
会阴
中极
石门
神阙
下脘
中脘
巨阙
中庭
玉堂
华盖
天突

任脉

Conception Vessel (Ren)

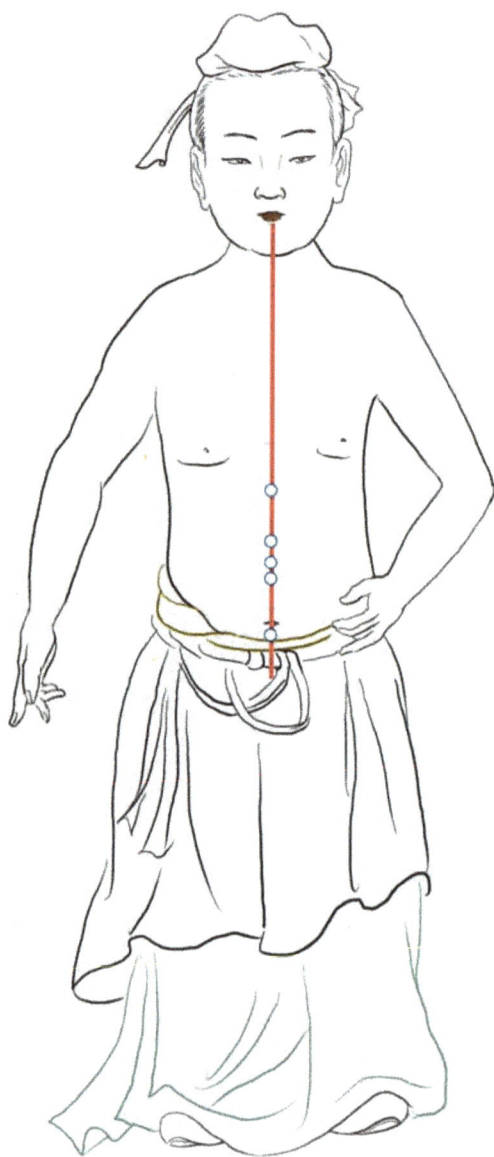

冲脉

Thoroughfare Vessel (Chong)

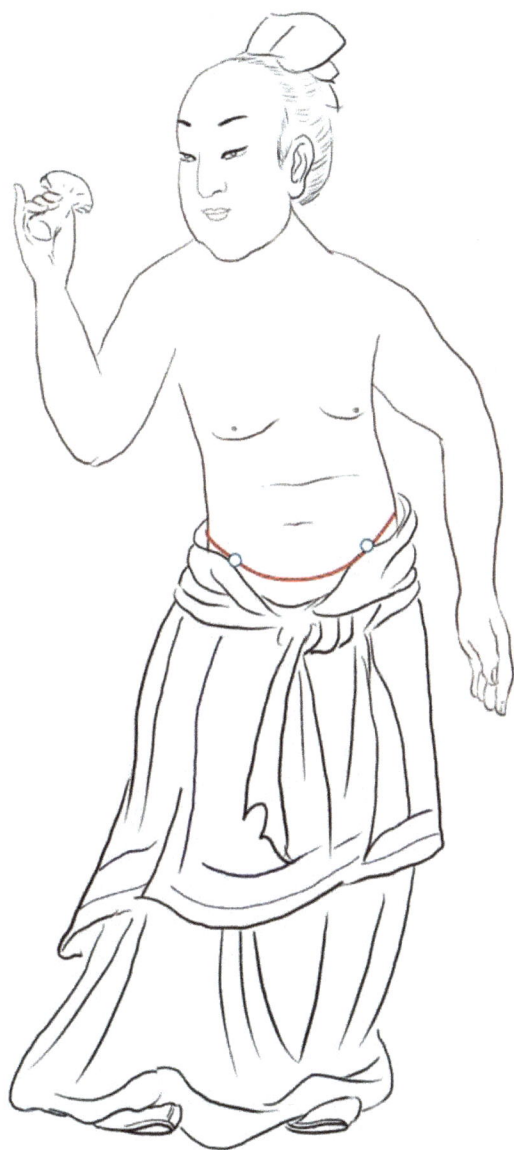

带脉

Belt Vessel (Dai)

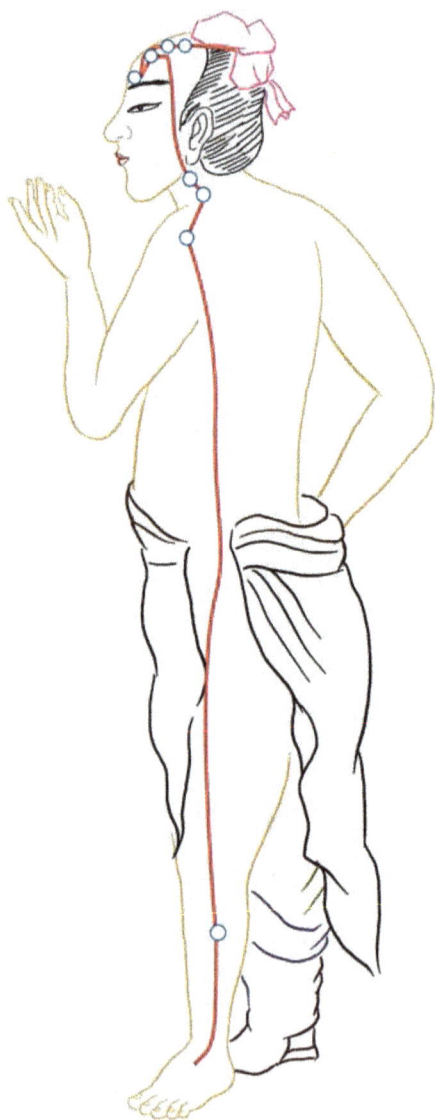

阳维脉

Yang Link Vessel (Yang Wei)

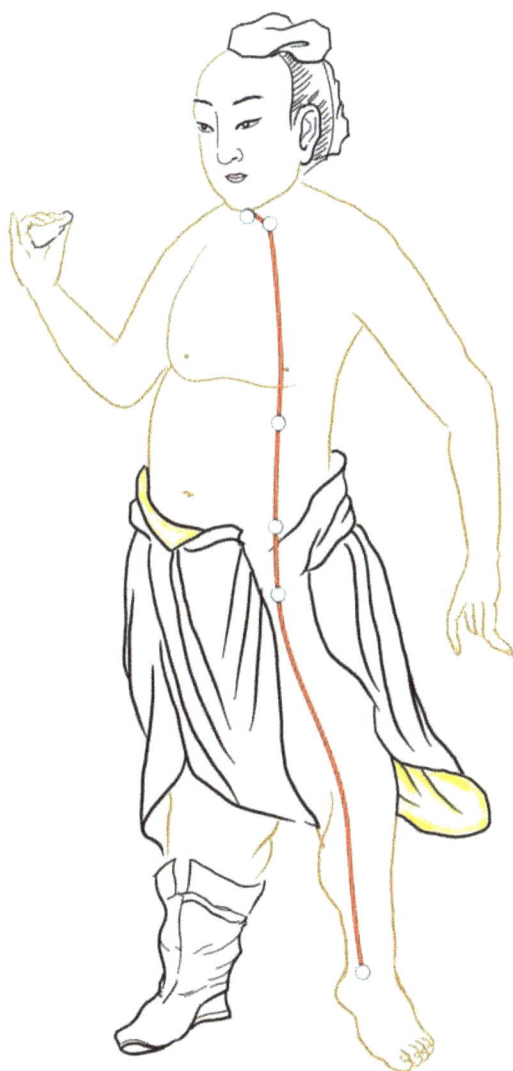

阴维脉

Yin Link Vessel (Yin Wei)

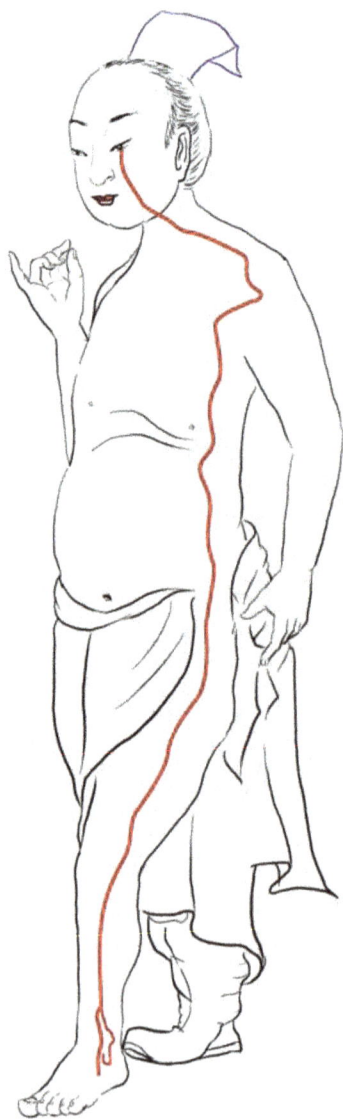

阳蹻脉

Yang Heel Vessel (Yang Qiao)